M000287090

THE PERFECT METABOLISM PLAN FOR WOMEN OVER 60

A Keto diet to restore your energy and regain your metabolism.

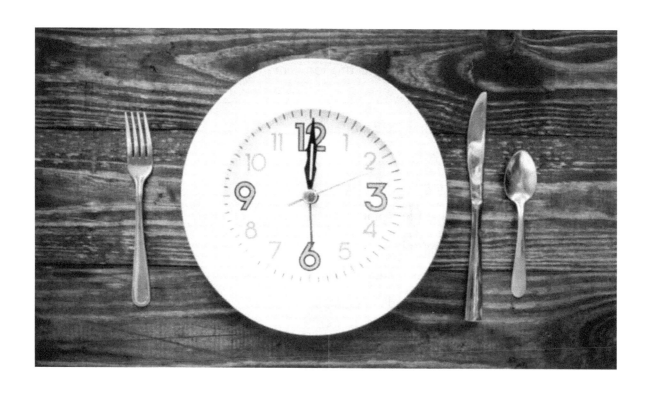

INTRODUCTION

The aim of this book is to provide you with the practical knowledge about the notion which is not only an abstraction based on philosophies but complete information which has been proven to stand the test of time.

This book is your short guide to intermittent fasting and the various processes involves in practicing intermittent Fasting. In the following pages, you will discover why even in this dispensation, the intermittent fasting guide is one great way to remain fit and be in shape even when you're above 60. Apart from keeping the body in shape, this practice has help curb lot of health issues and weakness in the body.

Intermittent Fasting can be a tool and a weapon. A deep understanding of this practice makes tremendous benefits available. Intermittent fasting can help improve our health, lose weight and also simplify our lifestyles. Learning this, regardless of your age, even above 60 may help you live longer.

Everybody today is searching for a way to be truly happy. This explains why we all find ourselves chasing after more money, more friends, and more stuff. Yet at the end of our lives, we realize that it was all for nothing. So, is the Stoic philosophy the best answer?

If you wish to learn more about stoicism, this eBook is perfect for you. The main goal of this book is to answer a lot of questions like what stoicism is, what is its history, what is its virtue and more.

It teaches how to become a better person by finding your inner peace and mindfulness. You needed a change, you wanted to get out of this circle, you wanted to succeed and now finally you found this book. Nobody is in charge of your life. It is only your responsibility to do all the steps towards better future. That is why you have to ask yourself honestly if you want to achieve something big and to inspire other people. If your answer is positive, then you have to stop wasting your time and implement exercises given in this book.

PART ONE

Chapter One: General Overview of the Keto-diet

What is the Keto-diet

The ketogenic diet is tied in with removing starches and eating more fats. Supporters infer 75% of their day by day calories from fat, 20 percent from protein and just 5 percent from starches. This is intended to initiate ketosis, a metabolic procedure wherein your cells need more sugars to use for vitality, so your body makes ketones and consumes fat. The inquiry is whether you are really getting yourself into a ketogenic state, or in case you're simply following a low-calorie, low-carb diet, which can likewise be viable. You're eating not many veggies, next to zero organic products, positively no grain items, a few meats yet very little. It's fundamentally a fat-based eating routine to arrive at a genuinely ketogenic state and look after it. It simply doesn't sound charming to most. On the off chance that ketosis is come to, it can prompt transient weight reduction. Be that as it may, the keto diet is amazingly prohibitive, making it difficult to follow and hard to keep up. "I think one about the greatest things is the manageability factor, is it something you can stay aware of, is it safe to stay aware of half a year or in about a year? I've seen it in a bunch of our patients, they attempt it for a month or two and shed pounds, and afterward they return three months and they have recaptured that weight in addition to more in light of the fact that it isn't manageable."

Advantages of Keto Diet

For certain reasons, individuals feel the keto diet is very horrendous which makes it a considerable amount testing to attempt particularly among the more established people. In any case, the keto diet wasn't made to work that way, the keto diet is only an eating plan that centers for the most part around nourishments that adds more to your solid fats and protein while radically decreasing the admission of starches to the least levels making it conceivable of achieving a larger number of calories from fats than from carbs. The keto-diet is known for its successful of radically lessening the weight of a person to them in including potential advantages in all. The following are advantages of keto-diet.

Increase in energy level.

In the initial days of this diet, it's normal for individuals to encounter the "keto flu," a concise period where you may have cerebral pains, exhaustion, perplexity, and sickness. These side effects are an indication that your body is changing from consuming glucose (sugar from carbs) for vitality to consuming fat, a procedure called ketosis. The changeover can leave you feeling drained for a day or two, yet once you get through to the fat-consuming stage, you may discover you have substantially more vitality and more prominent perseverance. "You can accomplish more without breaking the walls. At the point when we utilize fat as fuel, our perseverance improves and is increasingly practical.

Decrease in anxiety and tension

While these discoveries are starter, in one investigation of mice, the keto diet decreased nervousness. The exploration recommends this could be because of the defensive mind advantages of admission of healthy fats and low degrees of sugar. A subsequent report found that mice presented to a ketogenic diet while in utero demonstrated less weakness to nervousness and wretchedness than mice destined to moms who were not on the keto diet.

Protection against type 2 diabetes

The keto diet slices your everyday starches below 20 grams, for individuals with analyzed diabetes, this may assist them in dealing with the condition. A one-year study found that placing individuals with type 2 diabetes into ketosis drastically improved their glucose control.

The liver gets healthier

Fat amassing in the liver is ordinarily connected with prediabetes and type 2 diabetes. In genuine cases, greasy liver ailment can harm the liver. Specialists test for the condition by estimating levels of liver compounds utilizing blood tests. "These proteins were fundamentally diminished following one year in the clinical patients, demonstrating less danger of creating greasy liver illness. On the off chance that you've been told you're in danger for greasy liver, you might need to check out this eating regimen plan.

Enjoy profound rest

So many individuals on a ketogenic diet report resting a lot easier, says Pamela Ellgen, a fitness coach and creator of Sheet Pan Ketogenic. Be that as it may, during the alteration time frame (the initial three to five days after you start keto), you may encounter a sleeping disorder or trouble staying unconscious. This will end once your body acclimates to ketosis and consuming put away fat. At that point, you may discover you're ready to rest longer, rest further, and feel increasingly loose and rested when you wake up.

It helps treat cancer

Early research proposes that the keto diet may slow the development of carcinogenic tumors. "Cancer cells have a lot of insulin receptors on them, making them thrive in conditions high in glucose and insulin," says Brandon Olin, host of The Deskbound Podcast, which centers on conquering the harm of a stationary way of life. "It's basically giving malignant growth cells a wellspring of fuel to benefit from and develop." The examination recommends ketone bodies may give vitality to your body without taking care of the tumors.

Your cerebrum appears to be keener

While sugar might be an extraordinary speedy type of vitality, it doesn't keep your cerebrum at its best. There is a ton of proof turning out which recommends that the mind works more effectively on ketones than it does on glucose, however the examination is all genuinely new. Olin says. Ketones are made to fuel the mind without glucose. An enrolled dietitian and creator of The Ketogenic Diet. On an ordinary eating regimen, the mind gets 100 percent of its vitality from glucose. On a ketogenic diet, up to 66% of the cerebrum's vitality originates from ketones. It's justifiable that cerebrum capacity would change radically on a ketogenic diet.

Cautions for Keto

1. The "keto Flu"

"A few people report that when they start ketosis, they simply feel debilitated. They can once in a while be upchuck, gastrointestinal trouble, a ton of exhaustion, and laziness. This supposed keto flu for the most part goes following a couple of days. According to research, about 25% of individuals who attempt a keto diet experience these side effects, with exhaustion being the most widely recognized. "That happens in light of the fact that your body comes up short on sugar to consume for vitality, and it needs to begin utilizing fat. That change alone is sufficient to cause your body to feel tired for a couple of days."

However, you might have the option to limit the impacts of keto Flu by drinking a lot of water and getting a lot of rest. Axe, who sells keto-related enhancements on his site, additionally prescribes consolidating common vitality sources to fight exhaustion, as matcha green tea, natural espresso, or adaptogenic herbs.

2. Diarrhea

On the off chance that you wind up hurrying to the washroom all the more regularly while on a ketogenic diet, a snappy web search will give you that you're not the only one. This might be because of the gallbladder the organ that produces bile to assist break with bringing down fat in the eating regimen—feeling "overpowered," says Ax.

Loose bowels can likewise be because of an absence of fiber in the keto diet, says Kizer, which can happen when somebody reduces carbs (like entire grain bread and pasta) and doesn't enhance with other fiber-rich nourishments, similar to vegetables. It can likewise be brought about by a narrow mindedness to dairy or fake sugars things you may be eating a greater amount of since changing to a high-fat, low-carb way of life.

3. Diminished athletic performance

A few competitors depend on the ketogenic diet, for weight reduction as well as for improved performance in their game, also. Be that as it may, Edward Weiss, PhD, partner teacher of sustenance and dietetics at Saint Louis University doesn't get it. "I hear cyclists state constantly that they're quicker and better now that they're on the keto diet, and my first inquiry is, 'Well, how much weight did you lose?'" he says.

In an ongoing report in the Journal of Sports Medicine and Physical Fitness, Weiss and his associates found that members performed more awful on high-force cycling and pursuing undertakings four days on a ketogenic diet, contrasted with those who'd went through four days on a high-carb diet. Weiss says that the body is in a progressively acidic state when it's in ketosis, which may restrict its capacity to perform at top levels.

"Simply shedding a couple of pounds is sufficient to give you an enormous preferred position on the bicycle, however I'm worried that individuals are ascribing the advantages of weight reduction to something explicit in the ketogenic diet," Weiss proceeds. "In all actuality, the advantages of weight reduction could be at any rate in part counteracted by decreases in execution."

4. Ketoacidosis

On the off chance that you have type 1 or type 2 diabetes, you shouldn't follow the keto diet except if you have your primary care physician's authorization and close supervision, says Kizer. "Ketosis can really be useful for individuals who have hyperglycemia issues, however you must be aware of your glucose and check your glucose levels a few times each day," she says.

That is on the grounds that, for individuals with diabetes, ketosis can trigger a risky condition called ketoacidosis. This happens when the body puts away an excessive number of ketones—acids delivered as a side-effect of consuming fat—and the blood turns out to be excessively acidic, which can harm the liver, kidney and brain. Left untreated can be disastrous.

Ketoacidosis has additionally been accounted for in individuals without diabetes who were following low-carb eats less, in spite of the fact that this confusion is very uncommon. Side effects of ketoacidosis incorporate a dry mouth, visit pee, sickness, terrible breath, and breathing challenges; in the event that you experience these while following the keto diet, check in with a specialist immediately. These kinds of to and fro weight changes can add to confused eating, Kizer says, or can exacerbate an effectively undesirable relationship with nourishment. "I think the keto diet claims to individuals who have issues with divide control and with voraciously consuming food," she says. "Furthermore, much of the time, what they truly need is a way of life mentor or an expert advocate to assist them with finding a good pace of those issues."

Can Keto Have side effects

You've heard the expression "No Pain, No Gain" with regards to accomplishing objectives in the exercise center. A similar saying can likewise be utilized for viable weight control plans, in that you won't have the option to accomplish physical and psychological well-being objectives without investing the exertion and abandoning a large number of the decent things throughout everyday life. With regards to the keto diet, it's the same, and each diet that rolls out extraordinary improvements for the positive will bring about some symptoms as your body adjusts. The kinds of reactions can shift from individual to individual and rely upon many factors about your wellbeing and way of life. On the off chance that you've just found out about a portion of the reactions that accompany this extraordinary eating routine and are beginning to go crazy, don't freeze. We're going to separate all that you have to know with regards to what your body will encounter when utilizing these weight reduction items.

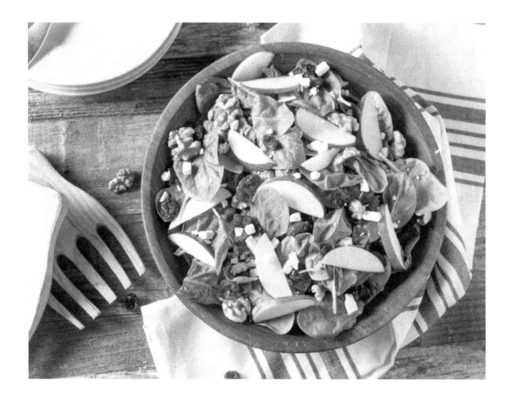

What happens in your body when you eat Keto

The keto diet is protected as long as you stick to explicit rules and ensure you don't keep your body from crucial supplements. While the reactions recorded on this page are normal, they are connected to your body's digestion rolling out some uncommon improvements. Much the same as setting off to the center for the principal couple of times after a languid nonappearance will cause a great deal of sore muscles and solidness, expelling certain things from your eating regimen will require some opportunity to change. You will likewise observe a great deal of reports that feature dangers of a keto diet, yet these for the most part do not have a ton of understanding into the reasons why so many individuals appear to experience the ill effects of these symptoms. We won't adulate it and enclose it by a bow to reveal to you that it will be a simple time. You ought to truly scrutinize any eating regimen that makes such guarantees. Rather, we expect to give all of you the data you have to ensure you lessen reactions to a base. Understanding the negatives that you may experience and why they happen will assist you with avoiding them through and through. What's more, with the correct supper plan and enhancements, you can maintain a strategic distance from the greater part of these inside and out.

Signs you're in Ketosis

At the point when you eat a low-starch ketogenic diet, your whole digestion shifts. Your glucose drops, your muscle versus fat consumes, and you begin delivering ketones that furnish your cerebrum and body with spotless, productive vitality. In any case, how would you know what ketosis side effects are and whether your new eating routine is working?

Except if you know the basic manifestations and symptoms of ketosis, it's not constantly evident when your body is making the fat-consuming movement into keto. Clearly, coming up next are plainly composed signs you are in ketosis. Ongoing keto advances a great deal of positive changes to your body and mind, from weight reduction to better vitality. It's these medical advantages that have made keto so mainstream.

1. Quick Weight Loss

You'll most likely lose noteworthy load in your first couple a long time of keto. It won't be all fat misfortune (that comes later). It'll for the most part be water weight that you lose when you consume your glycogen stores. Glycogen is your body's put away type of glucose (sugar). On keto, you needn't bother with a lot of it. At the point when you're in a calorie shortage on keto, your body goes to put away muscle versus fat. Glycogen is for the most part water — three particles of water for each atom of glucose — so when you consume your glycogen stores and don't top off them by eating carbs, you shed a few pounds of water weight

2. Supported Fat Loss

When you're a little while into keto, your glycogen stores will be gone and you'll begin consuming muscle to fat ratio. Here's the ticket:

- Low-carb, high-fat eating less junk food brings down your glucose levels
- Low glucose levels lessen your insulin levels.
- Low insulin signals fat consuming and ketone production. This fat-consuming state is the genuine driver of continued weight reduction on keto. The outcomes represent themselves:
- Women on keto lost more weight than ladies on high-carb calorie-restriction[*]
- Sixteen young people lost more weight following a low-sugar diet than a low-fat eating routine more than twelve weeks.
- A 24-week ketogenic diet improved body sythesis (less fat, more muscle) in fat individuals.

Try not to be disheartened if your weight reduction eases back down following a long time on keto. The underlying weight reduction was likely water. Fat misfortune comes straightaway, and it's progressively continuous yet it'll occur.

3. Diminished Cravings

When you're keto-adjusted, you'll likely discover you pine for less bites, desserts, and treats. That is on the grounds that a high-fat, low-carb diet diminishes hunger in a few diverse ways[*]:

- Lowering ghrelin, your yearning hormone

- Reducing neuropeptide Y, a craving trigger in your mind

- Boosting CCK, a peptide that causes you to feel full

    On the off chance that appetite feels less squeezing to you and you think that its anything but difficult to go 5-8 hours without nourishment or yearnings, there's a decent possibility you're in ketosis.

4. Increasingly Stable Energy

Keto shifts your digestion from sugar-consuming to fat-consuming, which takes glucose change and insulin off the table. On keto, your glucose remains reliably low and stable, which implies you don't get the vitality rollercoaster of sugar rushes and sugar crashes. Ketones are additionally an outstandingly proficient vitality source. Your mitochondria (the powerhouses of your cells) produce more vitality with less free radicals (provocative side-effects of digestion) when they consume ketones. In the event that you experience consistent, copious vitality for the duration of the day, chances are you've changed from consuming sugar to consuming fat for fuel.

Unwanted Signs You're in Ketosis

There are a lot of explored supported advantages to keto, yet getting into ketosis can accompany a couple of reactions. These includes;

1. Awful Breath

At the point when you begin consuming fat for fuel, one of the ketone bodies you produce is CH3)2CO. At the point when you're initially changing into keto, you may discharge CH3)2CO through your breath. It doesn't occur to everybody, except it tends to be a symptom of ketosis (called "keto breath").Acetone is the principle fixing in nail clean remover. It smells sweet, fruity, and somewhat like fuel. On the off chance that your breath smells that way, you're presumably delivering more CH3)2CO than expected as your body adjusts to keto. Fortunately keto breath as a rule leaves after you've been keto for half a month.

2. Keto Flu

Keto influenza portrays this season's cold virus like manifestations that originate from your body's progress from copying carbs to copying fat. It takes your body a couple of days to switch over, and during that time there's a ton going on with your science. Your kidneys start removing water and electrolytes as your glycogen stores drain. You regularly likewise get sugar and carb withdrawal, which feels like caffeine withdrawal.

3. Stomach related Problems

A few people experience stomach related pain in the main couple of long stretches of keto. The issue could be deficient fiber the inedible material that feeds gut microorganisms and animates solid defecations. At the point when you cut out carbs, you're likewise removing out numerous fiber-rich nourishments so make certain to supplant them with low-carb, stringy vegetables like kale, broccoli, and asparagus.

4. Muscle Cramps

In the event that you seize up on keto, don't freeze. The causes are likely simple to fix.

Muscle squeezes in keto are typically identified with lack of hydration and drained electrolytes.

Ensure you drink a lot of water and take a top notch electrolyte supplement with potassium, magnesium, and sodium.

5. Rest Issues

You may experience difficulty dozing during your keto progress. For the most part, this is a direct result of carb withdrawal. Sugar is physiologically addictive, and removing it causes withdrawal manifestations, one of which is a sleeping disorder. Your body may likewise be fighting the absence of carbs in your eating routine since it's trapped in limbo: it hasn't adjusted to consuming fat yet, yet it additionally doesn't have any carbs to use as a fuel source. Thus, your cerebrum can discharge cortisol between 2 a.m. to 4 a.m., guiding you to wake up and discover nourishment. Sleep deprivation as a rule settle following two or three weeks in keto, if not sooner. Meanwhile, you may try different things with melatonin a sheltered and successful regular rest supplement

What about Cholesterol? And other concerns about eating fat

•   The greatest impact on blood cholesterol level is the blend of fats and sugars in your eating routine not the measure of cholesterol you eat from nourishment.

•   Although it stays essential to restrain the measure of cholesterol you eat, particularly on the off chance that you have diabetes, for a great many people dietary cholesterol isn't as tricky as once accepted.

•   The body utilizes cholesterol as the beginning stage to make estrogen, testosterone, nutrient D, and other fundamental mixes.

• Cholesterol in the circulation system, explicitly the awful LDL cholesterol, is what's generally significant in deciding wellbeing hazard.

Know your macros and tracking after 60

Eating well is something beyond tallying calories. To genuinely have a decent eating routine, you must have an assortment of supplements that give your body vitality and help your stomach related framework work. The most ideal approach to watch what you're eating is, both to shed pounds or simply remain solid, to follow macronutrients. Doing that can assist you with arriving at your wellbeing and wellness objectives quicker than concentrating on calories alone.

Following macros over calories is useful for such a significant number of reasons. This strategy for nourishment logging can assist you with understanding which kinds of nourishment cause you to feel fortunate or unfortunate; which nourishments improve your athletic exhibition; and which food sources assist you with centering or make you drag. Tallying macros can likewise assist you with moving your present dietary patterns to more beneficial examples as long as possible.

You'll have to figure out how to peruse a nourishment realities name for this methodology, however the advantages far exceed the time you'll spend getting a handle on the idea of a full scale diet.

What are macronutrients?

Macronutrients are atoms we need in enormous sums, otherwise called the principle supplements we have to just endure. Micronutrients, interestingly, are substances required in a lot littler sums, for example, nutrients, minerals and electrolytes. The three macronutrients are starches, proteins and fats. Regardless of craze abstains from food, you do require each of the three: Cutting out any one macronutrient puts you in danger for supplement lacks and sickness.

Starches

Starches give you speedy vitality. At the point when you eat carbs, your body changes over them to glucose (sugar) and either utilizes that sugar quickly or stores it as glycogen for sometime in the future, regularly during exercise and in the middle of suppers. Complex sugars like dull vegetables and entire grains likewise advance stomach related wellbeing since they're high in dietary fiber.

Protein

Protein encourages you develop, fix wounds, assemble muscle and battle off diseases, to give some examples capacities. Proteins are made of amino acids, which are the structure squares of numerous structures in your body. You need 20 distinctive amino acids, nine of which are basic amino acids, which means your body can't create them all alone and you should get them from nourishment. High-protein nourishments incorporate poultry, meat, fish, soy, yogurt, cheddar and other dairy items. On the off chance that you stay with a plant-based eating routine, a few starches, vegetables and beans are likewise acceptable wellsprings of protein.

Fats

Dietary fat is required for your body to do its numerous employments. You need fat to ingest the fat-dissolvable nutrients (A, D, E and K), to protect your body during chilly climate and to go significant stretches of time without eating. Dietary fat additionally ensures your organs, bolsters cell development and instigates hormone creation.

What number of calories does each macronutrient have?

Each macronutrient relates to a particular calorie sum for every gram:

- Carbohydrates have four calories for every gram

- Proteins have four calories for every gram

- Fats have nine calories for every gram

What number of macros would it be a good idea for me to eat?

There's actually no response to this inquiry: Every individual is unique, and accordingly, every individual's ideal macronutrient admission will be extraordinary. Be that as it may, the government dietary proposals recommend this macronutrient proportion:

- 45 to 60 percent sugar

- 20 to 35 percent fats

- Remainder from protein

Step by step instructions to figure your macros

Presently you recognize what macros are and what number of calories they have. Next, you'll have to do some math. That is on the grounds that your admission proportion is written in rates however sustenance data is given in grams. I'll utilize my large scale admission for instance.

- First, you have to know what number of calories you eat (or need to eat) every day. I eat approximately 2,300 calories for every day.
- Next, decide your optimal proportion. I like to eat around 60 percent carbs, 25 percent fat and 25 percent protein.
- Then, increase your complete every day calories by your rates.
- Finally, separate your calorie sums by its calorie-per-gram number.
- Here's the way I would compute my calories for each macronutrient

Carbs: 2,300 x 0.60 equivalents 1,160. I eat 1,160 calories worth of carbs every day (hi, additional cut of toast).

Protein: 2,300 x 0.25 equivalents 575, so I get 575 calories worth of protein.

Fats: 2,300 x 0.25 equivalents 575. I additionally get 575 calories contained dietary fat.

To figure the real gram sums:

- Carbs (four calories for each gram): 1,160 separated by 4 equivalents 287.5 grams of carbs.

- Protein (four calories for every gram): 575 isolated by 4 equivalents 143.75 grams of protein

- Fat (nine calories for every gram): 575 isolated by 9 equivalents 63.8 grams of fat.

In the event that you don't care for math, don't worry. The web is home to a scope of macronutrient number crunchers that will figure it out for you. The best large scale adding machines

IIFYM

IIFYM means "In the event that It Fits Your Macros" an expression and well known hashtag utilized by the full scale following network to allude to their adaptable eating less junk food approach. This adding machine is one of the most thorough accessible. It gathers way of life and wellbeing data that numerous adding machines don't, for example, how dynamic you are grinding away, what sort of longings you have and whether you have any ailments.

Solid Eater

Solid Eater's large scale number cruncher computes your macronutrient proportion dependent on your age, sexual orientation, tallness, weight and action level. You can modify your proportion dependent on whether you need to diminish your weight, lose 10 percent muscle to fat ratio, keep up or put on weight. The full scale adding machine is quite okay, since you can see your proportion throughout the day, three dinners, four suppers or five suppers.

Tips on how to maintain good health after 60

Fifty is an extraordinary age, and it's an ideal time to begin concentrating on life span. The best guidance for anybody in their fifties is to utilize this decade to proactively address any medical problems you have and make an establishment for fifty additional long stretches of good wellbeing and joy.

From mentality to dietary patterns, there is an extraordinary arrangement you can do to improve your wellbeing and even turn around a portion of the harm previously done. Utilize this schedule as motivation. Essentially pick each or two things in turn to begin. The best changes to make for your life span are long haul way of life changes, so make the most of them!

Start a Healthy Lifestyle: Having a solid way of life can indicate 11 years to your life, however it's not generally as simple as it sounds. Start little.

Scientists saw individuals matured 45 and over and found that three components could signify 11 or 12 additional long periods of life. Individuals who (1) quit smoking, (2) ate heaps of products of the soil, and (3) expanded their activity lived longer. This was genuine regardless of whether they began these propensities in their 60s and past. Along these lines, begin adding a long time to your life today.

Lose the Extra Weight: Think there's no good reason for getting more fit in your 60s? Think the harm has just been finished? You are a long way from right. Getting in shape and setting up a solid way of life currently can do ponders for your wellbeing, particularly for your heart. Try not to blame your age; find a workable pace finding a good pace a sound weight now. You'll feel good and may even live more.

Get Tested: From malignant growth to coronary illness, on account of current medication, specialists can get things early and make a move, however just on the off chance that you give them a possibility. Converse with your primary care physician about your hazard factors and make certain to catch up on all the tests or screenings suggested for your age and clinical history. Without a doubt, screenings aren't fun, yet they can spare lives. Exercise is probably the best thing you can accomplish for your body. In addition to the fact that exercise helps assemble sound muscle, look after versatility, and keep the weight off, it improves your heart's wellbeing, keeps your psyche sharp, keeps up your equalization, and can even assistance keep up your sexual coexistence. It won't take long for you to find the entirety of the motivations to practice a few times each week (or more).

Ponder Aging: Having an inspirational demeanor toward maturing can really add a long time to your life. Actually, analysts found that a decent disposition about maturing could add 7.5 years to your life. That is an inconceivable number. Why the huge life span help? Nobody knows without a doubt. While there could be a connection between constructive reasoning and stress, specialists likewise feel that individuals with an uplifting mentality may make changes in practices that lead to a more drawn out life.

Increment in your Antioxidant Intake: What makes cancer prevention agents so incredible? They are what shield plants from the inconceivably harming impacts of the sun. Plants are presented to UV radiation throughout the day, which makes harm their cells. To shield from getting "seared" by this radiation, plants have grown high groupings of cancer prevention agents.

At the point when you eat plants, your body can utilize these equivalent cancer prevention agents to forestall harm to its own cells. It's phenomenal and simple. Discover which plants have the most noteworthy centralizations of cell reinforcements and eat a wide assortment of foods grown from the ground for the best impact.

Stay Energized: Being progressively dynamic encourages you live more and not as a result of the advantages of every day work out. Analysts inspected the calorie use of 300 individuals and found that the individuals who consumed the most calories in a day had a 32% decrease in the danger of death. Keeping yourself dynamic can do ponders for life span. Along these lines, shroud the remote (and the sofa), stroll as much as you can, and do whatever conceivable to keep dynamic and empowered consistently.

Learn New Things: Your cerebrum adores learning regardless of your age. The more new things it attempts to comprehend and the more associations it attempts to make, the better it capacities. Shake up your everyday practice by learning new things. Have you constantly needed to figure out how to cook? Maybe you need to figure out how to assemble something with your hands. Or on the other hand possibly you should simply change your day by day read to give your mind something new to consider.

Other than being intriguing, drawing in your cerebrum may decrease your hazard for Alzheimer's ailment and different types old enough related dementia—also, it'll make you all the more fascinating.

Grin: In all honesty, driving a grin all over can truly change your disposition. Your cerebrum gets signals from your face and thinks "Hello, we're grinning, something acceptable must occur."

Really soon your temperament really improves. Grinning can be an extraordinary method to lessen pressure. So make your 60s your grin decade and be more joyful and less pushed.

How aging affects your health

Recognizing what's in store and how to slow a portion of those progressions can enable you to remain as agreeable and dynamic as could reasonably be expected.

1. Heart

Your heart siphons the entire day and night, regardless of whether you are conscious or snoozing. It will siphon more than 2.5 billion beats during your lifetime! As you age, veins lose their versatility, greasy stores develop against supply route dividers and the heart needs to work more diligently to coursed the blood through your body. This can prompt (hypertension) and atherosclerosis (solidifying of the supply routes).

Dealing with your body with the correct sorts of fuel will assist you with keeping your heart solid and solid. You can deal with your heart by practicing and eating heart-sound nourishments.

2. Bones, Muscles and Joints

As we age, our bones shrivel and thickness. A few people really become shorter! Others are increasingly inclined to breaks on account of bone misfortune. Muscles, ligaments, and joints may lose quality and adaptability.

Exercise is an extraordinary method to slow or forestall the issues with bones, muscles and joints. Keeping up quality and adaptability will help keep you solid. Also, a solid eating routine including calcium can help your bones solid. Make certain to converse with your primary care physician about what sorts of diet and exercise are directly for you.

3. Stomach related System

Gulping and stomach related reflexes delayed down as we age. Gulping may get more enthusiastically as the throat contracts less powerfully. The progression of discharges that help digest nourishment in the stomach, liver, pancreas and small digestive system may likewise be diminished. The diminished stream may bring about stomach related problems that were absent when you were more youthful.

4. Kidneys and Urinary Tract

Kidneys may turn out to be less effective in expelling waste from the circulatory system on the grounds that your kidneys get littler as they lose cells as you age. Constant infections, for example, diabetes or hypertension can cause significantly more harm to kidneys.

Urinary incontinence may happen because of an assortment of wellbeing conditions. Changes in hormone levels in ladies and having a broadened prostate in men are contributing components that lead to urinary incontinence.

5. Cerebrum and Nervous System

As we age, we normally lose cells. This is even valid in the cerebrum. Memory misfortune happens on account of the quantity of synapses diminishes. The cerebrum can make up for this misfortune by expanding the quantity of associations between cells to safeguard mind work. Reflexes may back off, interruption is almost certain and coordination is influenced.

6. Eyes

There are numerous vision changes that happen as we age. We may require help seeing items that are nearer as our focal point solidifies. We may have a progressively troublesome time finding in low-light conditions, and hues might be seen in an unexpected way. Our eyes might be less equipped for creating tears and our focal points may get cloudier. Normal eye issues related with age incorporate waterfalls, glaucoma and macular degeneration.

7. Ears

Over the top clamor all through your lifetime can cause hearing misfortune as you age. Numerous more seasoned grown-ups experience issues hearing more shrill voices and sounds, inconvenience hearing in occupied spots and all the more every now and again gathering earwax.

8. Hair, Skin, and Nails

As you age, your skin turns out to be increasingly dry and fragile, which can prompt more wrinkles. The fat layer under the skin diminishes, which brings about less perspiring. This may appear to be something to be thankful for, however it makes you increasingly powerless to warm stroke and warmth depletion in the late spring. Hair and nails develop increasingly slow weak. Hair will thin and turn dark.

9. Weight

Diminishing degrees of physical action and an easing back digestion may add to weiigth gain.

Your body will most likely be unable to consume off the same number of calories as it once could, and those additional calories will wind up being put away as fat.

While you can't forestall maturing, you can set yourself up for the different impacts of maturing, both outside and inside the body.

Importance of keto for aging

The cerebrum is typically totally subject to glucose, however is equipped for utilizing ketones as another vitality source, as happens with delayed starvation or constant taking care of a ketogenic diet. Research has indicated that ketosis is neuroprotective against ischemic abuse in rodents. This survey centers around exploring the unthinking connects to neuroprotection by ketosis in the matured. Recuperation from stroke and other pathophysiological conditions in the matured is testing. Cerebral metabolic rate for glucose, cerebral blood stream, and the resistances against oxidative pressure are known to decay with age, recommending brokenness of the neurovascular unit. One instrument of neuroprotection by ketosis includes succinate-initiated adjustment of hypoxic inducible factor-1alpha (HIF1α) and its downstream consequences for mediator digestion.

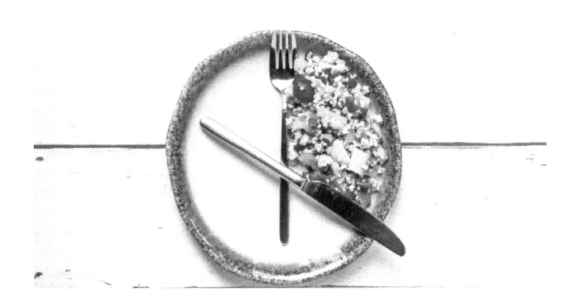

Chapter Two: Getting started with Keto, even after 60

As a woman who is above 60, might be considerably more keen on getting in shape than you were at 30. At this age, numerous ladies experience an easing back digestion at a pace of around 60 calories for every day. Easing back digestion combined with less exercise, strong degeneration and the potential for expanded desires can make it incredibly hard to control weight gain. There are many eating regimen choices accessible to help get thinner, yet the keto diet has been among the most well-known of late. We've gotten a great deal of inquiries around the viability of keto and how to comply with the eating regimen in a sound manner. Underneath, we have science-sponsored counsel that can give you the appropriate responses you're searching for on the off chance that you need to shed pounds on keto for women above than 60 years of age.

The distinction between the old and young woman during ketodiet

With regards to the keto diet versus a conventional eating regimen, tremendous contrasts exist between the prescribed recompenses for macronutrients, otherwise known as carbs, fat and protein. Also, the exceptionally advanced keto diet that is extremely popular today has key contrasts from the set up immovable epilepsy treatment for youngsters. Above all, the last is a recommended diet with close clinical supervision that is decisively determined to actuate ketosis while giving sufficient nourishment to forestall lack of healthy sustenance and advance typical development and improvement in youngsters. A ketogenic diet that is trailed by grown-ups most ordinarily for weight reduction and all the more as of late sort 2 diabetes the executives, yet additionally by certain competitors as a major aspect of their preparation routine is commonly not as absolutely determined as a ketogenic diet endorsed for youngsters with sedate safe epilepsy. The essential accentuation [of the grown-up keto diet is a decrease of starch admission to 20-60 grams for every day and restricting protein admission to 1.0-1.5 grams per kilogram of body weight or a perfect body weight if overweight to incite ketosis."

Troubleshooting

Investigating Keto: Get Back on Track and Maximize Your Results

The ketogenic diet keeps on developing in ubiquity. As research mounts with respect to its unmatched weight reduction potential, many are drawn towards the keto diet to acquire those outcomes for themselves. In any case, more than different weight control plans, keto can be requesting and a few people may level, seeing their outcomes come to a standstill. Find a portion of the more typical conditions that can stunt your advancement on the keto diet, and discover what you can do to get back headed straight toward your wellness objectives.

Ketosis and the Varying Degrees of Keto

The establishment of the ketogenic diet is to eat under 20-60 carbs every day so your liver produces ketones for your body to consume rather than glucose, which originates from sugar. While this idea appears to be sufficiently basic, there are really differing degrees of being keto-adjusted. For instance, keto strips frequently have eight hues that detail how profound into ketosis you are and keto blood screens will give you a rating that connotes your ketosis level.

Investigating Your Level of Ketosis

In case you're following the general rules of the keto diet and are experiencing difficulty moving beyond the most punctual phases of ketosis, your weight reduction progress will undoubtedly endure. On the off chance that that is the situation for you, at that point progressively definite activities might be required to get your body further into keto, or more keto-adjusted as it's frequently called. Look at these proposals for augmenting your keto progress and getting further into ketosis.

Is it true that you are Eating Enough Fats?

Since the keto diet confines you to simply veggies, meats, and dairy items, those aren't just recommendations. To get into a powerful phase of ketosis, it's urgent that you're expending enough fats. A lacking measure of either macronutrient can imperil your weight reduction potential, keeping you restricted to a low degree of ketosis. By and large, it's a decent dependable guideline that around 60-80% of your dietary admission should originate from an assortment of fats while on keto.

Is Your Protein Intake Moderate?

At the point when you're on keto, more protein isn't in every case better, yet inadequate sums can debilitate your ketosis too. Since most of your eating routine will comprise of great fats, protein is a similarly significant need, in spite of the fact that you don't require such a lot of protein as fat, notwithstanding. In case you're certain you're devouring enough fats however aren't advancing profound into ketosis, take a stab at expanding your protein admission and check whether that gets you back in fat-consuming mode.

Troubleshooting Digestive Problems on Keto

Fats require more vitality to process than some other sort of macronutrient, and they make up 60-80% of your dietary admission on keto.

In case you're experiencing difficulty adjusting to the higher admission of fats because of stomach related problems, it could cause issues like torment felt underneath the ribs and queasiness. Enhancing your eating regimen with the amino corrosive taurine can support your stomach related framework. Taurine is instrumental in the creation of bile and can help hugely with your absorption issue.

Trouble-shooting Heart Palpitations on Keto

One normal reaction that is habitually experienced on the ketogenic diet is heart palpitations. Basically, this implies your heart is thumping excessively quick, too delicately, or sporadically. The reasons for this can differ from mineral deficiency to absence of salt as your body adjusts to ketosis. Maintain a strategic distance from or limit heart palpitations by expanding your utilization of mineral-rich nourishments or enhancements. Likewise, since the incessant pee intrinsic in early periods of keto deny you of salt and water, expanding admission of those supplements can help too.

Troubleshooting Constipation on Keto

The issue of stoppage is no doubt because of an absence of fiber. While dairy and meat will in general make up most of nourishments eaten on the keto diet, neither of those nourishment types has adequate fiber. Since you won't eat high-fiber grains when you're on a keto diet, it's pivotal that you're devouring enough vegetables to keep your stomach related tract sound. In the event that you start to feel blocked up consistently when on keto, think about expanding your admission of high-fiber vegetables.

Keto Flu

As your body is adjusting to a ketogenic diet like Atkins20® or Atkins40®*, various changes may happen. These progressions are regularly alluded to as the "keto influenza." While these progressions aren't perilous, and generally die down following possibly 14 days, they can be awkward and badly designed. Beneath, we've illustrated some supportive tips to assist you with recognizing indications of keto influenza, fix bothersome keto influenza manifestations, and leap forward this progress while adhering to your eating routine.

What is Keto Flu?

At the point when your body starts to use fat, ketones are made. Ketones have a diuretic impact on your kidneys, which accelerates the measure of salt and water they process. This, for a few, may cause lack of hydration and an unevenness of electrolytes. Also, as sugar stores in the body start to exhaust and you change from a high carb to a low carb way of life—your body may start to feel distinctive in different manners.

Manifestations of Keto Flu

As each body is remarkable, you may encounter only a couple of side effects, or a blend of a few. You may even experience none! Keto influenza side effects may keep going for a couple of days, or for as long as about fourteen days.

Regular indications of keto influenza may include:

- Irritability

- Constipation

- Brain haze (or, the failure to think)

- Increased longings

- Headaches

- Nausea

- Muscle irritation and squeezing

- Dizziness

- Insomnia

Locate the Right Keto Flu Remedy for You

1.   Adjust your activity schedule: Light development may help muscle irritation and squeezing, however don't try too hard! Hurrying into another, serious exercise plan soon after redesigning your eating regimen may intensify manifestations.

2.   Hydrate: Increasing your water admission can soothe numerous keto influenza indications. Have a go at mixing your water with lemon or cucumber for an additional lift.

3.   Up your electrolytes: Electrolytes are significant minerals like sodium, potassium, and magnesium, and a few people can encounter a lack as their body changes with a ketogenic diet. In any case, be careful with sugary electrolyte substitution drinks! Attempt some full-salt juices.

4.   Foundation vegetables: Many keto-accommodating vegetables—like beets, cauliflower, broccoli, and verdant greens—are loaded with fiber and significant minerals, and may help any issues of stoppage or squeezing.

Physiological Insulin Resistance

Insulin is a significant hormone that controls numerous real procedures.

Be that as it may, issues with this hormone are at the core of numerous cutting edge wellbeing conditions.

Insulin obstruction, in which your cells quit reacting to insulin, is fantastically normal. Truth be told, over 32.2% of the U.S. populace may have this condition (1Trusted Source).

Contingent upon the indicative criteria, this number may ascend to 44% in ladies with heftiness and over 80% in some patient gatherings. About 33% of kids and young people with corpulence may have insulin opposition too

Insulin nuts and bolts

Insulin is a hormone emitted by your pancreas. Its fundamental job is to direct the measure of supplements coursing in your circulation system. Despite the fact that insulin is for the most part involved in glucose the executives, it additionally influences fat and protein digestion. At the point when you eat a feast that contains carbs, the measure of glucose in your circulatory system increments. The cells in your pancreas sense this expansion and discharge insulin into your blood. Insulin at that point goes around your circulation system, advising your cells to get sugar from your blood. This procedure brings about decreased glucose levels. Particularly high glucose can have poisonous impacts, making serious mischief and conceivably driving demise if untreated. Be that as it may, cells now and then quit reacting to insulin effectively. This is called insulin obstruction. Under this condition, your pancreas delivers considerably more insulin to bring down your glucose levels. This prompts high insulin levels in your blood, named hyperinsulinemia. After some time, your cells may turn out to be progressively impervious to insulin, bringing about an ascent in both insulin and glucose levels.

In the long run, your pancreas may get harmed, prompting diminished insulin creation. After glucose levels surpass a specific limit, you might be determined to have type 2 diabetes. Insulin opposition is the fundamental driver of this normal illness that effects about 9% of individuals around the world.

The most effective method to know whether you're insulin safe. Professional can utilize a few techniques to decide whether you're insulin safe. For instance, high fasting insulin levels are solid pointers of this condition. A genuinely exact test called HOMA-IR gauges insulin opposition from your glucose and insulin levels.

There are likewise approaches to gauge glucose control all the more straightforwardly, for example, an oral glucose-resistance test yet this takes a few hours. Your danger of insulin obstruction increments enormously in the event that you have overabundance weight or stoutness, particularly on the off chance that you have a lot of stomach fat. A skin condition called acanthosis nigricans, which includes dim spots on your skin, can in like manner show insulin opposition. Having low HDL (great) cholesterol levels and high blood triglycerides are two different markers unequivocally connected with this condition Insulin opposition is a sign of two regular conditions metabolic disorder and type 2 diabetes. Metabolic disorder is a gathering of hazard factors related with type 2 diabetes, coronary illness, and different issues. It's occasionally called insulin opposition disorder, as it's firmly connected to this condition.Its manifestations incorporate high blood triglycerides, circulatory strain, tummy fat, and glucose, just as low HDL (great) cholesterol levels. You might have the option to forestall metabolic disorder and type 2 diabetes by halting the advancement of insulin opposition.

Relationship to heart wellbeing

Insulin opposition is firmly connected with coronary illness, which is the main source of death over the globe. Indeed, individuals with insulin opposition or metabolic disorder have up to a 93% more serious danger of coronary illness.

Numerous different sicknesses, including non-alcoholic greasy liver malady (NAFLD), polycystic ovarian disorder (PCOS), Alzheimer's illness, and disease, are connected to insulin obstruction also

Approaches to lessen insulin opposition

It's genuinely simple to lessen insulin opposition. Strikingly, you can regularly totally turn around this condition by changing your way of life in the accompanying manners:

- Exercise. Physical action might be the single most effortless approach to improve insulin affectability. Its belongings are practically prompt.

- Lose stomach fat. It's vital to focus on the fat that collects around your primary organs by means of activity and different techniques.

- Stop smoking. Tobacco smoking can cause insulin opposition, so stopping should support.

- Reduce sugar consumption. Attempt to diminish your admission of included sugars, particularly from sugar-improved refreshments.

- Eat well. Eat an eating routine dependent on entire, natural nourishments. Incorporate nuts and greasy fish.

- Omega-3 unsaturated fats. These fats may diminish insulin opposition, just as lower blood triglycerides.

- Supplements. Berberine may improve insulin affectability and diminish glucose. Magnesium enhancements might be useful, as well (45Trusted Source, 46Trusted Source).

- Sleep. Some proof recommends that poor rest causes insulin opposition, so improving rest quality should support.

- Reduce stress. Attempt to deal with your feelings of anxiety on the off chance that you effectively get overpowered. Contemplation might be especially useful (48Trusted Source, 49Trusted Source).

- Donate blood. Significant levels of iron in your blood are connected to insulin opposition. For men and postmenopausal ladies, giving blood may improve insulin affectability.

- Intermittent fasting. Following this eating example may improve insulin affectability.

The majority of the propensities on this rundown likewise happen to be related with acceptable wellbeing, a long life, and security against sickness.

All things considered, it's ideal to counsel your wellbeing specialist about your choices, as different clinical medications can be compelling also.

Acne

Skin inflammation is a skin condition that happens when your hair follicles become stopped with oil and dead skin cells. It frequently causes whiteheads, zits or pimples, and typically shows up on the face, temple, chest, upper back and shoulders. Skin break out is generally basic among youngsters, however it influences individuals everything being equal.

Successful medicines are accessible, yet skin inflammation can be determined. The pimples and knocks recuperate gradually, and when one starts to leave, others appear to manifest.

Contingent upon its seriousness, skin inflammation can cause passionate misery and scar the skin. The prior you start treatment, the lower your danger of such issues.

Skin break out signs and manifestations change contingent upon the seriousness of your condition:

- Whiteheads (shut stopped pores)

- Blackheads (open stopped pores)

- Small red, delicate knocks (papules)

- Pimples (pustules), which are papules with discharge at their tips

- Large, strong, agonizing bumps underneath the outside of the skin (knobs)

- Painful, discharge filled bumps underneath the outside of the skin (cystic sores)

Indications.

Cystic skin break out

Skin break out signs and side effects shift contingent upon the seriousness of your condition:

- Whiteheads (shut stopped pores)

- Blackheads (open stopped pores)

- Small red, delicate knocks (papules)

- Pimples (pustules), which are papules with discharge at their tips

- Large, strong, difficult knots underneath the outside of the skin (knobs)

- Painful, discharge filled knots underneath the outside of the skin (cystic injuries)

When to see a specialist

In the event that self-care cures don't clear your skin inflammation, see your essential consideration specialist. The individual can endorse more grounded meds. On the off chance that skin inflammation endures or is serious, you might need to look for clinical treatment from a specialist who has practical experience in the skin (dermatologist).

For some ladies, skin break out can persevere for a considerable length of time, with flares basic seven days before period. This kind of skin inflammation will in general clear up without treatment in ladies who use contraceptives.

In more established grown-ups, an abrupt beginning of serious skin inflammation may flag a basic infection requiring clinical consideration.

The Food and Drug Administration (FDA) cautions that some mainstream nonprescription skin break out moisturizers, chemicals and other skin items can cause a genuine response. This kind of response is very uncommon, so don't mistake it for the redness, disturbance or irritation where you've applied drugs or items.

Look for crisis clinical assistance if in the wake of utilizing a skin item you experience:

- Faintness

- Difficulty relaxing

- Swelling of the eyes, face, lips or tongue

- Tightness of the throat

Causes

Four fundamental variables causes skin inflammation:

- Excess oil creation

- Hair follicles stopped up by oil and dead skin cells

- Bacteria

- Excess action of a sort of hormone (androgens)

Skin inflammation normally shows up all over, brow, chest, upper back and shoulders in light of the fact that these territories of skin have the most oil (sebaceous) organs. Hair follicles are associated with oil organs.

The follicle divider may lump and produce a whitehead. Or on the other hand the attachment might be available to the surface and obscure, causing a clogged pore. A zit may seem as though soil stuck in pores. In any case, really the pore is clogged with microorganisms and oil, which turns dark colored when it's presented to the air.

Pimples are raised red spots with a white community that create when blocked hair follicles become kindled or tainted with microscopic organisms. Blockages and aggravation that grow somewhere inside hair follicles produce cystlike bumps underneath the outside of your skin. Different pores in your skin, which are the openings of the perspiration organs, aren't typically engaged with skin inflammation.

Hazard factors for skin inflammation include:

• Age. Individuals of any age can get skin break out, however it's generally normal in adolescents.

• Hormonal changes. Such changes are normal in young people, ladies and young ladies, and individuals utilizing certain prescriptions, including those containing corticosteroids, androgens or lithium.

• Family history. Hereditary qualities assumes a job in skin inflammation. On the off chance that the two guardians had skin break out, you're probably going to create it, as well.

• Greasy or slick substances. You may create skin inflammation where your skin comes into contact with sleek moisturizers and creams or with oil in a work region, for example, a kitchen with fry tanks.

• Friction or weight on your skin. This can be brought about by things, for example, phones, cellphones, head protectors, tight collars and knapsacks.

• Stress. Stress doesn't cause skin inflammation, yet in the event that you have skin break out as of now, it might aggravate it.

Constipation

Constipation is one of the most widely recognized stomach related issues in the United States, influencing around 2.5 million. It's characterized as having hard, dry defecations, or going less than three times each week.

Causes

Your colon's primary employment is to assimilate water from remaining nourishment as it's going through your stomach related framework. It at that point makes stool (squander).

The colon's muscles inevitably drive the loss out through the rectum to be dispensed with. On the off chance that stool stays in the colon excessively long, it can turn out to be hard and hard to pass. Less than stellar eating routine as often as possible causes clogging. Dietary fiber and satisfactory water admission are important to help keep stools delicate.

Fiber-rich nourishments are commonly produced using plants. Fiber comes in dissolvable and insoluble structures. The solvent fiber can disintegrate in water and makes a delicate, gel-like material as it goes through the stomach related framework.

Insoluble fiber holds the vast majority of its structure as it experiences the stomach related framework. The two types of fiber get together with stool, expanding its weight and size while additionally relaxing it. This makes it simpler to go through the rectum.

Stress, changes in schedule, and conditions that moderate muscle constrictions of the colon or defer your desire to go may likewise prompt clogging.

Reasons

- low-fiber diet, especially counts calories high in meat, milk, or cheddar

- dehydration

- lack of activity

- delaying the motivation to have a defecation

- travel or different changes in schedule

- certain prescriptions, for example, high calcium stomach settling agents and agony drugs.

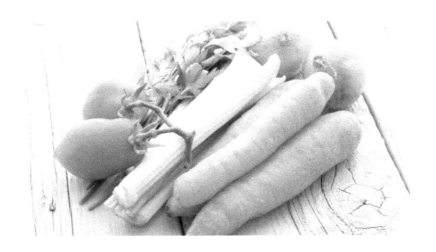

Who is in danger of Constipation?

Eating a less than stellar eating routine and not practicing are significant hazard factors for clogging. You may likewise be at more serious hazard in case you're:

•   Age 65 or more seasoned. More established grown-ups will in general be less truly dynamic, have hidden illnesses, and eat less fortunate eating regimens.

•   Confined to bed. The individuals who have certain ailments, for example, spinal rope wounds, regularly experience issues with solid discharges.

•   A lady or kid. Ladies have more successive scenes of obstruction than men, and youngsters are influenced more regularly than grown-ups.

•   Pregnant. Hormonal changes and weight on your digestion tracts from your developing infant can prompt stoppage.

How is it analyzed?

Numerous individuals influenced by stoppage decide to self-treat by changing their weight control plans, expanding activity, or utilizing over-the-counter intestinal medicines.

Be that as it may, diuretics shouldn't be utilized for over about fourteen days without counseling a doctor. Your body can get subject to them for colon work.

You should converse with your essential consideration supplier if:

•   You've had stoppage for over three weeks

•   You have blood in your stool

•   You experience stomach pain

•   You're encountering torment during solid discharges

•   You're getting in shape

•   You have abrupt changes in your defecations

Your PCP will pose inquiries about your indications, clinical history, and any meds or basic conditions.

A physical assessment may incorporate a rectal test and blood tests to check your blood tally, electrolytes, and thyroid capacity.

In extreme cases, extra tests might be required to recognize the reason for your indications. Tests may incorporate the accompanying:

Marker study

A marker study, likewise called a colorectal travel study, is utilized to test how nourishment is traveling through your colon. For this test, you'll swallow a pill that contains little markers that will appear on a X-beam.

Various stomach X-beams will be assumed control throughout the following scarcely any days so the specialist can envision how the nourishment is traveling through your colon and how well your intestinal muscles are functioning.

You may likewise be approached to eat an eating regimen high in fiber during the test.

Anorectal manometry

An anorectal manometry is a test used to assess butt-centric sphincter muscle work. For this test, your primary care physician will embed a flimsy cylinder with an inflatable tip into your rear-end.

At the point when the cylinder is inside, the specialist will blow up the inflatable and gradually haul it out. This test permits them to gauge your butt-centric sphincter's muscle quality and check whether your muscles are contracting appropriately.

Barium bowel purge X-beam

A barium purification X-beam is a kind of test used to look at the colon. For this test, you'll drink a unique fluid the night prior to the test to clear out the entrail.

The genuine test includes the addition of a color called barium into your rectum, utilizing a greased up tube. The barium features the rectum and colon territory, permitting the specialist to all the more likely view them on a X-beam.

Colonoscopy

A colonoscopy is another sort of test specialists use to analyze the colon. Right now, specialist will analyze your colon utilizing a cylinder that is furnished with a camera and light source.

A narcotic and torment drug is regularly given, so you'll likely not by any means recollect the assessment and should feel no agony.

To plan for this test, you'll be on a fluid eating regimen for 1 to 3 days, and you may need to take a diuretic or purification the night prior to the test to clear out the entrail.

Step by step instructions to treat and forestall obstruction

Changing your eating regimen and expanding your physical movement level are the most effortless and quickest approaches to treat and forestall stoppage. Attempt the accompanying procedures too:

•   Every day, drink 1/2 to 2 quarts of unsweetened, decaffeinated liquids, similar to water, to hydrate the body.

•   Limit utilization of liquor and jazzed drinks, which cause lack of hydration.

•   Add fiber-rich nourishments to your eating regimen, for example, crude foods grown from the ground, entire grains, beans, prunes, or wheat oat. Your day by day admission of fiber ought to be somewhere in the range of 20 and 35 grams.

•   Cut down on low-fiber nourishments, for example, meat, milk, cheddar, and prepared nourishments.

• Aim for around 160 minutes of moderate exercise each week, with an objective of 30 minutes out of each day in any event five times each week. Take a stab at strolling, swimming, or biking.

• If you want to have a defecation, don't delay. The more you pause, the harder your stool can turn into.

• Add fiber enhancements to your eating routine if necessary. Simply make sure to drink a lot of liquids since liquids assist fiber with working all the more effectively.

• Use intestinal medicines sparingly. Your PCP may endorse diuretics or purifications for a brief timeframe to help mollify your stools. Never use intestinal medicines for over about fourteen days without conversing with your primary care physician. Your body can get subject to them for appropriate colon work.

• Consider adding probiotics to your eating regimen, similar to those found in yogurt and kefir with live dynamic societies. StudiesTrusted Source have demonstrated that this dietary change can be useful for those with incessant blockage.

In the event that you despite everything experience difficulty with obstruction, your primary care physician may endorse prescriptions to help.

Dragon's breath

Dragon's Breath is a solidified pastry produced using grain plunged in fluid nitrogen. At the point when set in the eater's mouth, it produces fumes which leave the nose and mouth, giving the sweet its name. Dragon's Breath is made utilizing brilliant oat balls depicted as having a flavor like Froot Loops. The oat is plunged in fluid nitrogen and served in a cup. The eater utilizes a stick to stick the balls. Once in the eater's mouth, the cold of the fluid nitrogen consolidates with the glow of the mouth to discharge unmistakable fumes out of the nose and mouth. Dragon's Breath is noted for the scene of its utilization more than its flavor, with a few productions remarking on its similarity with Integra patterns

Scalp issues: Dandruff, Itchiness

With regards to dandruff, a great number of people center on the drops. Tingling, then again, might be the most awkward reaction. So what precisely is your scratchy scalp attempting to let you know? The following are the most well-known side effects of dandruff and approaches to get your scalp solid once more.

Indications and causes

Drops and an irritated, flaky scalp are the principle side effects of dandruff. White, slick pieces commonly aggregate in your hair and on your shoulders and frequently deteriorate throughout the fall and winter months, when the air is dry.

Pinpointing the specific reason for your irritated, flaky scalp can be troublesome, yet here are a couple of regular guilty parties:

Bothered and slick skin, a condition otherwise called seborrhea dermatitis (an increasingly extreme type of dandruff) not shampooing enough, which causes skin cells to gather and make chips and tingling Yeast called malassezia, which exasperate your scalp and cause overabundance skin cell development

distinctive individual consideration items may cause contact dermatitis, which makes your scalp red and irritated. Men create dandruff more as often as possible than ladies. Individuals who will in general have oilier hair or live with specific ailments, (for example, Parkinson's sickness or HIV) are likewise at higher hazard. You may have begun to see indications around pubescence, however dandruff can create at any age.

So what's your bothersome scalp attempting to let you know? Coming up next are four basic answers.

1. Not all shampoos are the equivalent

On the off chance that your scalp is bothersome, you might have the option to get some alleviation by utilizing over-the-counter (OTC) shampoos that are planned to help with dandruff.

Getting the correct fit may take some experimentation, so in the event that you haven't had karma before, attempt once more. At times rotating at least two cleanser types can likewise help.

A few items you may see on the racks include:

Head and Shoulders and Jason Dandruff Relief contain zinc pyrithione, which is antibacterial and antifungal. Dandruff isn't brought about by growth, yet it despite everything helps by easing back the creation of overabundance skin cells.

Neutrogena T/Gel is a tar-based cleanser. Coal can ease conditions from dandruff to psoriasis by easing back how rapidly your scalp's skin cells kick the bucket and drop off. This kind of cleanser can stain hair, so be cautious in case you're blonde or dark.

Neutrogena T/Sal has a portion of salicylic corrosive and may reduce the measure of scale you have. They can leave your scalp dry, nonetheless. On the off chance that you find that your scalp is especially dry, ensure you catch up with a saturating conditioner.

Selsun Blue has the intensity of selenium sulfide. It can slow your skin cells from passing on and furthermore lessen malassezia. This sort of cleanser may likewise stain lighter shades of hair.

Nizoral is a ketoconazole cleanser, which means it contains an expansive range antifungal. You can discover this sort of wash OTC or by solution.

On the off chance that you don't realize which to pick, approach your primary care physician for a proposal. To get dandruff leveled out, you may need to utilize extraordinary cleanser when you do cleanser (ideal recurrence differs dependent on hair type).

When things are leveled out, you may just need to utilize the cleanser incidentally to keep up great impact.

2. Saturate

A dry scalp will in general chip and tingle, yet as a rule the drops you'll involvement in dry skin are littler and less sleek. Reestablishing dampness to the scalp can help with irritation.

The best cream may as of now be perched on your kitchen rack. Coconut oil has saturating and antibacterial properties, making it an incredible, regular decision for battling dryness.

3. Practice great cleanliness and quit scratching!

Shampooing regularly enough can keep oils under control, assisting with dandruff manifestations. While you are grinding away, attempt to fight the temptation to scratch your scalp. The irritation is at first brought about by bothering from dandruff, however scratching will build aggravation and lead to an endless loop.

Utilizing such a large number of items in your hair can bother the scalp and lead to more irritation. Take a stab at disposing of anything extra from your own consideration routine and adding back in gradually to find which gels, showers, and different items don't exacerbate your side effects.

4. You have to unwind

Stress can exasperate or even exacerbate dandruff for certain people. While malassezia isn't acquainted with your scalp by pressure, it can flourish if your invulnerable framework is undermined, which is actually what stress does to your body.

Help your scalp out and unwind. Take a stab at going for a helpful stroll or rehearsing yoga. You may even think that its supportive to keep a log of unpleasant occasions. Record what they are and how they sway your dandruff. That way, you can put forth a valiant effort to maintain a strategic distance from potential triggers later on.

Lowered alcohol Tolerance

On the off chance that your resistance rises, and you drink increasingly more to get a similar impact you once got from one glass of wine, at that point you could be going into perilous ground. Fortunately, on the off chance that you think your resilience is rising, retaliating is straightforward: simply offer your body a reprieve from liquor with some liquor free days every week. For the vast majority, you can 'reset' your entire framework by having an alcohol or liquor free period. Furthermore, individuals feel better for it. I can tell when they stroll through the entryway by their facial appearance. The thing that matters is sensational. Once you've reset your resilience you won't need as much alcoholic drink to feel the impact.

Elevated Cholesterol

Cholesterol is a waxy substance found in your blood. Your body needs cholesterol to fabricate solid cells, yet significant levels of cholesterol can build your danger of coronary illness.

With elevated cholesterol, you can create greasy stores in your veins. In the end, these stores develop, making it hard for enough blood to move through your supply routes. Now and again, those stores can break out of nowhere and structure a coagulation that causes a cardiovascular failure or stroke.

Elevated cholesterol can be acquired, however it's frequently the consequence of unfortunate way of life decisions, which make it preventable and treatable. A sound eating regimen, normal exercise and at times drug can help lessen elevated cholesterol.

Indications

Elevated cholesterol has no indications. A blood test is the best way to recognize on the off chance that you have it.

Hazard factors

Variables that can build your danger of terrible cholesterol incorporate.

Horrible eating routine: Eating immersed fat, found in creature items, and trans fats, found in some industrially heated treats and saltines and microwave popcorn, can raise your cholesterol level. Nourishments that are high in cholesterol, for example, red meat and full-fat dairy items, will likewise expand your cholesterol.

Weight: Having a weight file (BMI) of 30 or more noteworthy puts you in danger of elevated cholesterol.

Absence of activity: Exercise helps support your body's HDL, or "acceptable," cholesterol while expanding the size of the particles that make up your LDL, or "awful," cholesterol, which makes it less unsafe.

Smoking: Cigarette smoking harms the dividers of your veins, making them progressively inclined to collect greasy stores. Smoking may likewise bring down your degree of HDL, or "great," cholesterol.

Age: Because your body's science changes as you age, your danger of elevated cholesterol climbs. For example, as you age, your liver turns out to be less ready to evacuate LDL cholesterol.

Diabetes: High glucose adds to more significant levels of risky cholesterol called low-thickness lipoprotein (VLDL) and lower HDL cholesterol. High glucose likewise harms the coating of your supply routes.

Difficulties

Improvement of atherosclerosis: High cholesterol can cause a hazardous gathering of cholesterol and different stores on the dividers of your corridors (atherosclerosis). These stores (plaques) can diminish blood course through your supply routes, which can cause difficulties, for example,

Chest torment. On the off chance that the veins that supply your heart with blood (coronary courses) are influenced, you may have chest torment (angina) and different manifestations of coronary conduit sickness.

Respiratory failure. On the off chance that plaques tear or crack, a blood coagulation can frame at the plaque-burst site — obstructing the progression of blood or breaking free and stopping a supply route downstream. On the off chance that blood stream to part of your heart stops, you'll have a respiratory failure.

Stroke. Like a respiratory failure, a stroke happens when a blood coagulation squares blood stream to part of your mind.

Avoidance

A similar heart-sound way of life changes that can bring down your cholesterol can help keep you from having elevated cholesterol in any case. To help forestall elevated cholesterol, you can:

Eat a low-salt eating regimen that accentuates natural products, vegetables and entire grains

Farthest point the measure of creature fats and utilize great fats with some restraint

Lose additional pounds and keep up a solid weight

- Stop smoking
- Exercise on most days of the week for at any rate 30 minutes
- Savor liquor balance, if by any means
- Oversee pressure

Hair Loss

This can influence only your scalp or your whole body. It very well may be the consequence of heredity, hormonal changes, ailments or prescriptions. Anybody can encounter hair loss, yet it's increasingly regular in men. Hairlessness ordinarily alludes to inordinate male pattern baldness from your scalp. Genetic male pattern baldness with age is the most well-known reason for hair loss. A few people want to let their male pattern baldness run its course untreated and unhidden. Others may cover it up with hairdos, cosmetics, caps or scarves. What's more, still others pick one of the medications accessible to forestall further balding and to reestablish development.

Side effects

- Male-design hair sparseness
- Female-design hair sparseness
- Inconsistent loss of hair (alopecia areata)
- Footing alopecia

The loss of hair can show up from various perspectives, contingent upon what's causing it. It can come on out of nowhere or step by step and influence only your scalp or your entire body. A few kinds of hair loss are transitory, and others are changeless. The Signs and side effects may include:

Progressive diminishing on head. This is the most widely recognized kind of male pattern baldness, influencing the two people as they age. In men, hair frequently starts to retreat from the temple in a line that takes after the letter M. Ladies ordinarily hold the hairline on the temple however have a widening of the part in their hair.

Roundabout or sketchy bare spots. A few people experience smooth, coin-sized bare spots. This kind of male pattern baldness for the most part influences only the scalp, yet it now and then additionally happens in facial hair or eyebrows. At times, your skin may get irritated or excruciating before the hair drops out.

Unexpected relaxing of hair. A physical or enthusiastic stun can make hair release. Bunches of hair may turn out when brushing or washing your hair or much after delicate pulling. This kind of male pattern baldness as a rule causes in general hair diminishing and not bare patches.

Full-body male pattern baldness. A few conditions and clinical medications, for example, chemotherapy for malignant growth, can bring about the loss of hair all over your body. The hair typically becomes back.

Patches of scaling that spread over the scalp. This is an indication of ringworm. It might be joined by broken hair, redness, growing and, now and again, overflowing.

Causes

Individuals regularly lose around 100 hairs every day. This generally doesn't cause perceptible diminishing of scalp hair on the grounds that new hair is developing in simultaneously. Male pattern baldness happens when this pattern of hair development and shedding is upset or when the hair follicle is crushed and supplanted with scar tissue. Balding is commonly identified with at least one of the accompanying elements:

Family ancestry (heredity): The most widely recognized reason for male pattern baldness is a genetic condition called male-design hairlessness or female-design sparseness. It as a rule happens step by step with maturing and in unsurprising examples a subsiding hairline and bare spots in men and diminishing hair in ladies.

Hormonal changes and ailments: An assortment of conditions can cause perpetual or brief male pattern baldness, including hormonal changes because of pregnancy, labor, menopause and thyroid issues. Ailments incorporate alopecia -reata which causes sketchy male pattern baldness, scalp contaminations, for example, ringworm and a hair-pulling issue called trichotillomania.

Meds and enhancements: Balding can be a reaction of specific medications, for example, those utilized for malignant growth, joint inflammation, melancholy, heart issues, gout and hypertension.

Radiation treatment to the head: The hair may not develop back equivalent to it was previously.

An extremely distressing occasion: Numerous individuals experience a general diminishing of hair a while after a physical or passionate stun. This kind of male pattern baldness is transitory.

Insomania

A sleeping disorder is a rest issue in a difficult situation falling and, or staying unconscious.

The condition can be present moment (intense) or can keep going quite a while (incessant). It might likewise go back and forth.

Intense a sleeping disorder endures from 1 night to half a month. A sleeping disorder is incessant when it occurs in any event 3 evenings per week for 3 months or more.

Types

There are basically two types of sleeping disorder also known as insomnia and these includes;

The primary: This implies your rest issues aren't connected to some other wellbeing condition or issue.

The secondary: This implies you experience difficulty dozing in view of a wellbeing condition (like asthma, discouragement, joint inflammation, malignant growth, or acid reflux); torment; medicine; or substance use (like liquor).

Causes

The primary includes:

•   Stress identified with enormous life occasions, similar to an occupation misfortune or change, the passing of a friend or family member, separate, or moving

•   Things around you like clamor, light, or temperature

•   Changes to your rest plan like stream slack, another move busy working, or negative behavior patterns you got when you had other rest issues

The secondary includes

Emotional wellness issues like discouragement and nervousness

•   Medications for colds, hypersensitivities, misery, hypertension, and asthma

•   Pain or inconvenience around evening time

•   Caffeine, tobacco, or liquor use

•   Hyperthyroidism and other endocrine issues

•   Other rest issue, similar to rest apnea or fretful legs disorder

A sleeping disorder Risk Factors

A sleeping disorder influences ladies more than men and more seasoned individuals more than more youthful ones. Youthful and middle-age African Americans additionally have a higher hazard.

Other hazard factors include:

- Long-term disease

- Mental medical problems

- Working night moves or moves that turn

- Insomnia Symptoms

- Symptoms of a sleeping disorder include:

- Sleepiness during the day

- Fatigue

- Grumpiness

- Problems with focus or memory

A sleeping disorder Diagnosis

Your PCP will do a physical test and get some information about your clinical history and rest history.

They may instruct you to save a rest journal for up to 14 days, monitoring your rest examples and how you feel during the day. They may converse with your bed accomplice about how much and how well you're dozing. You may likewise have uncommon tests at a rest place.

Sleeping disorder Treatment

Intense a sleeping disorder may not require treatment.

In the event that it's difficult for you to do ordinary exercises since you're worn out, your PCP may endorse resting pills for a brief timeframe. Medications that work rapidly yet quickly can assist you with staying away from issues like sleepiness the following day.

Try not to use over-the-counter resting pills for sleep deprivation. They may have symptoms, and they will in general work less well after some time.

For incessant a sleeping disorder, you'll need treatment for the conditions or medical issues that are keeping you alert. Your primary care physician may likewise recommend conduct treatment. This can assist you with changing the things you do that exacerbate a sleeping disorder and realize what you can do to advance rest.

Sleep deprivation Complications

Our bodies and cerebrums need rest so they can fix themselves. It's likewise essential for learning and keeping recollections. In the event that a sleeping disorder is keeping you alert, you could have:

- A higher danger of medical issues like hypertension, heftiness, and despondency

- A higher danger of falling, in case you're a more seasoned lady

- Trouble centering

- Anxiety

- Grumpiness

- Slow response time that can prompt a fender bender

Sleep deprivation Prevention

- Good rest propensities, likewise called rest cleanliness, can assist you with beating sleep deprivation. Here are a few hints:

- Go to rest simultaneously every night, and find a good pace same time every morning. Make an effort not to take rests during the day, since they may make you less drowsy around evening time.

- Don't use telephones or digital books before bed. Their light can make it harder to nod off.

- Avoid caffeine, nicotine, and liquor late in the day. Caffeine and nicotine are energizers and can shield you from nodding off. Liquor can make you wake up in the center of the night and hurt your rest quality.

- Get standard exercise. Make an effort not to turn out near sleep time, since it might make it difficult to nod off. Specialists propose practicing at any rate 3 to 4 hours before bed.

- Don't eat a substantial feast late in the day. However, a light nibble before sleep time may enable you to rest.

- Make your room agreeable: dim, calm, and not very warm or excessively cold. In the event that light is an issue, utilize a dozing cover. To conceal sounds, attempt earplugs, a fan, or a background noise.

- Follow a daily practice to unwind before bed. Peruse a book, tune in to music, or scrub down.

- Don't utilize your bed for something besides rest and sex.

- If you can't nod off and aren't lazy, find a workable pace something quieting, such as perusing until you feel tired.

- If you will in general falsehood alert and stress over things, make a daily agenda before you hit the hay. This may assist you with setting your interests aside for the evening.

keto rash

In the event that you've been engaged with the wellbeing and health world recently, you've likely known about the keto diet. The ketogenic diet, additionally alluded to as the keto diet, is a low-carb, high-fat eating routine. With an extremely low starch admission, the body can run on ketones from fat rather than glucose from carbs. This prompts expanded fat-consuming and weight reduction.

Be that as it may, likewise with any uncommon dietary change, there can be some undesirable reactions. Starting reactions of the keto diet may incorporate cerebrum mist, exhaustion, electrolyte unevenness, and even a keto rash. Right now will get all that you have to think about the keto rash, including what can cause it, how to treat it, and how to keep it from occurring.

Manifestations of the keto-rash

Keto rash, regularly officially known as prurigo pigmentosa, is an uncommon, fiery state of the skin portrayed by a red, irritated rash around the storage compartment and neck.

The keto rash is a kind of dermatitis that can happen in anybody yet is generally basic in Asian ladies. A large portion of the top to bottom research regarding the matter has recently included youthful Japanese ladies. The indications of keto-rash incorporate;

- An irritated, red rash that happens essentially on the upper back, chest, and guts

- Red spots, called papules, that take on a web-like appearance

- A dull dark colored example left on the skin once the spots vanish

Reasons for the keto rash

Research on the connection between the keto diet and prurigo pigmentosa is restricted. Nonetheless, some proof recommends a relationship between's the two. Analysts are as yet not so much sure what causes keto rash, however there are believed to be a few related conditions. These include:

- Still's ailment

- Sjögren's disorder

- H. pylori disease

Furthermore, there's a solid relationship between's this intense rash and the nearness of ketosis, which is the manner by which it gets its epithet "keto rash."

Ketosis happens most generally because of prohibitive abstaining from excessive food intake and can likewise be found in diabetics. On the off chance that ketosis is joined by uncontrolled sugars, it can prompt a hazardous condition known as ketoacidosis. With the keto diet, the objective is to be in ketosis.

Hazard factors

- A number of components can expand your danger of male pattern baldness, including:

- Family history of thinning up top, in both of your parent's families

- Age

- Significant weight reduction

- Certain ailments, for example, diabetes and lupus

- Stress

Anticipation

- Most sparseness is brought about by hereditary qualities (male-design hairlessness and female-design hairlessness). This sort of male pattern baldness isn't preventable.

- These tips may assist you with keeping away from preventable sorts of male pattern baldness:

- Avoid tight haircuts, for example, meshes, buns or braids.

- Avoid enthusiastically turning, scouring or pulling your hair.

- Treat your hair delicately when washing and brushing. A wide-toothed brush may help forestall pulling out hair.

- Avoid brutal medications, for example, hot rollers, hair curlers, hot oil medicines and permanents.

- Avoid drugs and enhancements that could cause male pattern baldness.

- Protect your hair from daylight and different wellsprings of bright light.

- Stop smoking. A few examinations show a relationship among smoking and hair sparseness in men.

Adapted but not feeling right

It's quite usual to not feel right with keto, these feelings as somewhat usual but as times goes on, you will get used to this method and this will slay all doubts, making you adapted to this technique.

Chapter Three EATING KETO – Simple Keto Recipes

What you'll be eating and not eating

On the off chance that quick weight reduction while expending about boundless measures of fat sounds unrealistic, "reconsider," keto diet fans state. Supporters of the stylish high-fat, low-carb feast plan swear it clears the mind while bringing down the number on the scale.

Albeit long haul wellbeing impacts of the eating routine, which requires generally 80% of your every day calories to originate from fat, are as yet obscure for the normal individual, the Keto diet has for quite some time been utilized to treat youngsters with epilepsy and individuals with diabetes. Yet, the greatest inquiry of everything is how does eating keto diet nourishments cause you to get in shape when you're eating bacon, margarine, and cheddar? Continue perusing for the subtleties, in addition to realize which nourishments you can (and can't!) eat on this eating routine.

Carbs (5-10% of calories)

Estimated grams of carbs every day dependent on a 2,000-calorie diet: 40

"Definitely constraining your admission of glucose, the typical vitality hotspot for your cells, diminishes insulin emissions in your body. Since low degrees of glucose are coming in, the body utilizes what is put away in the liver and afterward the muscles," says Rania Batayneh, MPH, the creator of The One Diet: The Simple 1:1:1 Formula for Fast and Sustained Weight Loss. After around three or four days, the entirety of the amassed is spent.

"For an elective wellspring of vitality, your liver will begin to change over fat into ketones, which will at that point be discharged into the circulatory system and be utilized by your phones for vitality. Essentially, your mind and muscles will be filled by fat rather than sugars," says Michelle Hyman, MS, RD, CDN an enlisted dietitian at Simple Solutions Weight Loss.

Nosh on noodles or other high-carb nourishments and you'll send your body once again into glucose-consuming mode; eat nearly nothing and you'll likely feel your vitality hauling. Most keto health food nuts expect to eat between 20 to 60 grams of carbs every day to keep up that ketone-consuming state called "ketosis."

You should expect to score your carbs from high-fiber, water-rich foods grown from the ground to normally help hydration and keep your stomach related framework murmuring along. Uncertain of whether a produce pick is low in carbs? Reach for alternatives become over the ground (verdant greens, peppers, and stalk-molded vegetables), as opposed to subterranean (root veggies like potatoes, carrots, and parsnips), as they normally offer less carbs.

Genuine instances of carb keto diet nourishments:

- Tomatoes

- Eggplant

- Asparagus

- Broccoli

- Cauliflower

- Spinach

- Green Beans

- Cucumber

- Bell peppers

- Kale

- Zucchini

- Celery

- Brussels grows

- Protein (10-20% of calories)

Protein is basic to fabricate muscle cells and consume calories. Eat excessively or excessively little of it as a major aspect of your keto diet nourishment plan and you'll wind up subverting your objectives.

Without carbs and protein, for example, in case you're adhering to the low-carb share of keto and eating more fat and less protein than suggested, your body will go to muscle tissue as fuel. This, thus, will bring down your general bulk and the quantity of calories you consume very still.

Overdose on protein (following this macronutrient breakdown, that would liken to anything well beyond one six-ounce steak and one four-ounce chicken bosom) and you'll put undue strain on your kidneys. Additionally, your body will change over the abundance protein to starches for fuel. That is the specific inverse objective of the keto diet.

Go for around 15% of calories from high-fat protein sources like those underneath. A few, for example, Greek yogurt, eggs, and cheddar, give significant nutrients to keep your hair, eyes, and invulnerable framework solid.

"While prepared meats like frankfurter and bacon are in fact allowed on the keto diet, I'd prescribe to constraining them since they're high in sodium," Hyman says.

Genuine instances of protein keto diet nourishments:

- Chicken, dim meat if conceivable

- Turkey, dim meat if conceivable

- Venison

- Beef

- Salmon

- Sardines

- Tuna

- Shrimp

- Pork

- Lamb

- Eggs

- Natural cheeses

- Unsweetened, entire milk plain Greek yogurt

- Whole milk ricotta cheddar

- Whole milk curds

- Opt for natural, field raised, and grass-took care of, if conceivable, for meat and poultry

Fat (70-80% of calories)

Surmised grams of carbs every day dependent on a 2,000-calorie diet: 165

Here's the place the majority of your admission becomes possibly the most important factor. A few examinations have demonstrated that a higher-fat eating routine can decrease desires and levels of hunger animating hormones ghrelin and insulin.

At the point when you're amassing your keto diet nourishment stash, go full-fat. Furthermore, don't worry over the dietary cholesterol content, a factor of how a lot of creature protein you eat, recommends an investigation distributed in The Journal of Nutrition. Rather, center around expending a higher proportion of unsaturated fats (flaxseed, olive oil, nuts) to soaked fats (fat, red meat, palm oil, spread). Since you're devouring a larger part of calories from fat, it's significant to concentrate on filling up with choices that are more averse to stop up your corridors and less inclined to build your disease hazard.

Genuine instances of fat keto diet nourishments:

- Olive oil

- Avocado oil

- Olives

- Avocados

- Flaxseeds

- Chia seeds

- Pumpkin seeds

- Sesame seeds

- Hemp hearts

- Coconuts

- Nuts

- Natural, no-sugar-included nut spreads

What to Avoid

Make it simpler to remain inside the macronutrient system of the keto diet by avoiding these nourishments;

- Beans, peas, lentils, and peanuts

- Grains, for example, rice, pasta, and oats

- Low-fat dairy items

- Added sugars and sugars

- Sugary refreshments, including juice and pop

- Traditional nibble nourishments, for example, potato chips, pretzels, and wafers

- Most natural products, aside from lemons, limes, tomatoes, and little segments of berries

- Starchy vegetables, including corn, potatoes, and peas

- Trans fats, for example, margarine or other hydrogenated fats

- Most alcohols, including wine, brew, and improved mixed drinks

Keto power food

The ketogenic diet has become very well known as of late. Studies have discovered this low-carb, high-fat eating regimen is compelling for weight reduction, diabetes and epilepsy. There's likewise early proof to show that it might be helpful for specific malignant growths, Alzheimer's sickness and different illnesses, as well. A ketogenic diet regularly constrains carbs to 20–60 grams for each day. While this may appear to be testing, numerous nutritious nourishments can without much of a stretch fit into along these lines of eating. The following are solid nourishments to eat on a ketogenic diet.

1. Fish

Fish and shellfish are very keto-accommodating nourishments. Salmon and other fish are plentiful in B nutrients, potassium and selenium, yet for all intents and purposes without carb. Be that as it may, the carbs in various sorts of shellfish differ. For example, while shrimp and most crabs contain no carbs, different sorts of shellfish do. While these shellfish can in any case be remembered for a ketogenic diet, it's imperative to represent these carbs when you're attempting to remain inside a restricted range. Here are the carb means 3.5-ounce (100-gram) servings of some mainstream kinds of shellfish.

- Clams: 5 grams

- Mussels: 7 grams

- Octopus: 4 grams

- Oysters: 4 grams

- Squid: 3 grams

Salmon, sardines, mackerel and other greasy fish are exceptionally high in omega-3 fats, which have been found to bring down insulin levels and increment insulin affectability in overweight and fat individuals.

Likewise, visit fish admission has been connected to a diminished danger of malady and improved psychological wellness.

Intend to devour at any rate two servings of fish week after week.

2. Low-Carb Vegetables

Non-bland vegetables are low in calories and carbs, yet high in numerous supplements, including nutrient C and a few minerals.

Vegetables and different plants contain fiber, which your body doesn't process and ingest like different carbs.

In this way, take a gander at their edible (or net) carb check, which is complete carbs short fiber.

Most vegetables contain not very many net carbs. In any case, devouring one serving of "bland" vegetables like potatoes, yams or beets could put you over your whole carb limit for the afternoon.

The net carb mean non-boring vegetables ranges from under 1 gram for 1 cup of crude spinach to 8 grams for 1 cup of cooked Brussels grows.

Vegetables likewise contain cancer prevention agents that help secure against free radicals, which are flimsy atoms that can cause cell harm. In addition, cruciferous vegetables like kale, broccoli and cauliflower have been connected to diminished malignancy and coronary illness chance.

Low-carb veggies make incredible substitutes for higher-carb nourishments. For example, cauliflower can be utilized to copy rice or pureed potatoes, "zoodles" can be made from zucchini and spaghetti squash is a characteristic substitute for spaghetti.

3. Cheddar

Cheddar is both nutritious and tasty.

There are many sorts of cheddar. Luckily, every one of them are low in carbs and high in fat, which makes them an incredible fit for a ketogenic diet. One ounce (28 grams) of cheddar gives 1 gram of carbs, 7 grams of protein and 20% of the RDI for calcium. Cheddar is high in immersed fat, yet it hasn't been appeared to build the danger of coronary illness. Truth be told, a few investigations recommend that cheddar may help ensure against coronary illness. Cheddar likewise contains conjugated linoleic corrosive, which is a fat that has been connected to fat misfortune and upgrades in body structure. Likewise, eating cheddar normally may help decrease the loss of bulk and quality that happens with maturing. A 12-week study in more established grown-ups found that the individuals who expended 7 ounces (210 grams) of ricotta cheddar every day experienced increments in bulk and muscle quality through the span of the investigation.

4. Avocados

Avocados are unbelievably sound.

3.5 ounces (100 grams), or around one-portion of a medium avocado, contain 9 grams of carbs.

Be that as it may, 7 of these are fiber, so its net carb check is just 2 grams.

Avocados are high in a few nutrients and minerals, including potassium, a significant mineral numerous individuals may not get enough of. In addition, a higher potassium admission may help make the progress to a ketogenic diet simpler. Moreover, avocados may help improve cholesterol and triglyceride levels.

5. Meat and Poultry

Meat and poultry are viewed as staple nourishments on a ketogenic diet.

Crisp meat and poultry contain no carbs and are plentiful in B nutrients and a few minerals, including potassium, selenium and zinc.

They're additionally an extraordinary wellspring of top notch protein, which has been appeared to assist save with muscling mass during a low-carb diet. One examination in more established ladies found that devouring an eating regimen high in greasy meat prompted HDL cholesterol levels that were 8% higher than on a low-fat, high-carb diet. It's ideal to pick grass-took care of meat, if conceivable. That is on the grounds that creatures that eat grass produce meat with higher measures of omega-3 fats, conjugated linoleic corrosive and cell reinforcements than meat from grain-took care of creatures.

Keto Food shopping list

Setting off to the supermarket is a hard enough errand without the additional work of looking for explicit things since you're sticking to a specific nourishment plan. In case you're following the keto diet, exploring the passageways looking for things that the high-fat, low-carb way of life permits can be significantly trickier. So what are a portion of the things you need to ensure discover their way into your truck? Indeed, the accompanying rundown will make following this arrangement as simple as opening your cooler.

Canned Sardines

High in omega-3 unsaturated fats and a top notch wellspring of protein, canned sardines are a scrumptious keto staple. In addition, Mancinelli calls attention to that they likewise regularly come canned in olive oil, giving a solid portion of fat. She includes: "And they're prepared to eat a case that couple of keto nourishments can make!" Toss a couple on that fiery serving of mixed greens you're chipping away at, and presto: that is a keto-accommodating supper.

Salmon

On the other hand, if the simple thought of sardines causes you to flinch, salmon is an attractive other option. "Greasy fish are a significant commitment to any eating regimen due to their exceptionally high omega-3 fat substance. This is particularly imperative to a ketogenic health food nut who gets the vast majority of their calories from fat," Mancinelli says, including that other greasy fish alternatives incorporate mackerel and fish.

All around marbled Steak

When looking for meat, Mancinelli proposes searching for all around marbled cuts, similar to a ribeye or a NY strip. What's more, the explanation behind this one is truly straightforward: "When you're eating a ketogenic diet, it's regularly difficult to get enough fat and abstain from indulging protein." That way, she includes, you'll have the option to eat a littler bit of meat in light of the fact that the fat all through the slice will add to your sentiment of totality. Other well-known protein sources on the keto diet incorporate sheep, chicken, venison, turkey, fish, cod and, you got it.

Sweetners
Following a ketogenic diet includes decreasing high-carb nourishments like starches, pastries and prepared snacks.This is fundamental to arriving at a metabolic state called ketosis, which makes your body start separating fat stores rather than carbs to create vitality. Ketosis likewise requires diminishing sugar utilization, which can make it trying to improve refreshments, prepared merchandise, sauces and dressings. Luckily, there are different low-carb sugars that

you can appreciate. Here are the best sugars for a low-carb keto diet and some you ought to maintain a strategic distance from.

1. Stevia

Stevia is a characteristic sugar got from the Stevia rebaudiana plant.

It's viewed as a nonnutritive sugar, which implies that it contains next to zero calories or carbs. In contrast to customary sugar, creature and human examinations have demonstrated that stevia may assist lower with blooding sugar levels. Stevia is accessible in both fluid and powdered frame and can be utilized to improve everything from beverages to pastries.

Nonetheless, on the grounds that it's a lot better than customary sugar, plans require less stevia to accomplish a similar flavor. For each cup (200 grams) of sugar, substitute just 1 teaspoon (4 grams) of powdered stevia.

2. Sucralose

Sucralose is a counterfeit sugar that isn't utilized, which means it goes through your body undigested and in this way doesn't give calories or carbs. Splenda is the most widely recognized sucralose-put together sugar with respect to the market and famous on the grounds that it does not have the severe taste found in numerous other counterfeit sugars. While sucralose itself is sans calorie, Splenda contains maltodextrin and dextrose, two carbs that supply around 3 calories and 1 gram of carbs in every bundle. In contrast to different sorts of sugars, sucralose is anything but a reasonable substitute for sugar in plans that require preparing.

A few examinations have discovered that sucralose could create unsafe mixes when presented to high temperatures. Rather, use sucralose as a low-carb approach to improve beverages or nourishments like oats and yogurt and stick to different sugars for preparing. Splenda can be fill in for sugar in a 1:1 proportion for most plans. Be that as it may, unadulterated sucralose is multiple times better than normal sugar, so you'll just need to utilize a minor sum instead of sugar for your preferred nourishments.

3. Erythritol

Erythritol is a sort of sugar liquor a class of normally happening exacerbates that invigorate the sweet taste receptors on your tongue to impersonate the flavor of sugar. It's up to 80% as sweet as normal sugar, yet it contains just 5% of the calories at simply 0.2 calories per gram.

Moreover, however erythritol has 4 grams of carbs per teaspoon (4 grams), considers show that it might assist lower with blooding sugar levels in your body. Besides, because of its littler sub-atomic weight, it commonly doesn't cause the stomach related problems related with different kinds of sugar alcohols.

Erythritol is utilized in both heating and cooking and can be fill in for sugar in a wide assortment of plans. Remember that it will in general have a cooling mouthfeel and doesn't break up just as sugar, which can leave nourishments with a marginally lumpy surface. For best outcomes, swap around 1/3 cups (267 grams) of erythritol for each cup (200 grams) of sugar.

4. Xylitol

Xylitol is another kind of sugar liquor normally found in items like without sugar gum, confections and mints.

It's as sweet as sugar however contains only 3 calories for each gram and 4 grams of carbs per teaspoon (4 grams). However, as other sugar alcohols, the carbs in xylitol don't consider net carbs, as they don't raise glucose or insulin levels to the degree sugar does. Xylitol can be effortlessly added to tea, espresso, shakes or smoothies for a low-carb kick of flavor. It additionally functions admirably in heated merchandise yet may require a touch of additional fluid in the formula, as it will in general retain dampness and increment dryness. Since xylitol is as sweet as normal sugar, you can trade it for sugar in a 1:1 proportion.

Note that xylitol has been related with stomach related issues when utilized in high dosages, so downsize your admission on the off chance that you notice any unfriendly impacts.

5. Priest Fruit Sweetener

As its name suggests, priest organic product sugar is a characteristic sugar removed from the priest natural product, a plant local to southern China. It contains regular sugars and mixes called mogrosides, which are cell reinforcements that represent a great part of the sweetness of the organic product. Contingent upon the convergence of mogrosides, priest natural product sugar can be anyplace between 100–260 times better than normal sugar. Priest natural product extricate contains no calories and no carbs, making it an extraordinary choice for a ketogenic diet. The mogrosides may likewise invigorate the arrival of insulin, which can improve the transportation of sugar out of the circulatory system to help oversee glucose levels. Make certain to check the fixings name when purchasing priest organic product sugar, as priest natural product extricate is some of the time blended in with sugar, molasses or different sugars that can adjust the absolute calorie and carb content. Priest organic product sugar can be utilized anyplace you would utilize ordinary sugar. The sum you use can change between various brands dependent on what different fixings might be incorporated. While some suggest subbing utilizing an equivalent measure of priest organic product sugar for sugar, others inform slicing the sum concerning sugar down the middle.

Alcohol

In case you're following a ketogenic diet, you likely realize that high-carb treats are beyond reach. Yet, would you be able to drink alcohol while keto? Well, The answer is yes. Be that as it may, there are sure mixed beverages you should maintain a strategic distance from in case you're hoping to remain in ketosis. Drinking while at the same time following a keto diet can likewise have some unforeseen reactions. This is what you should think about drinking liquor in case you're keto. As a matter of first importance, you can drink liquor and remain in ketosis. Be that as it may, there's a trick. Despite the fact that one glass of something solid won't take your body out of ketosis, drinking liquor while following a keto diet will influence your advancement. In particular, it will hinder your pace of ketosis. When you drink, you'll keep on creating ketones and will stay in ketosis. In any case, your body treats ethanol (for example liquor) as a poison and will work to dispose of it.

"The liver will begin to process liquor as fast as could be expected under the circumstances, which implies it is utilized by the body before every single other supplement, including fat, so it eases back the way toward changing over unsaturated fats to ketones."

Drinking liquor won't eradicate all your advancement, yet it will affect ketosis. Some mixed beverages are starch bombs, while others are moderately keto-accommodating. Wine is a well-known liquor decision for those on the keto diet. Le Vin Parfait/Flickr With regards to remaining in ketosis, not every alcoholic choice is equivalent. "The short form: wine is lower in carbs than brew, so the vast majorities who eat keto pick wine. Unadulterated spirits like bourbon and vodka contain zero carbs, yet look out for sweet beverages – they may contain monstrous measures of sugar," prompted Andreas Eenfeldt, MD, by means of Diet Doctor. In case you're hoping to enjoy a liquor refreshment while adhering to a keto diet, select lower carb drink alternatives and keep away from over-the-top mixed drinks. Alcohol with 40% liquor by volume (80 proof) or higher will regularly have 0 grams net carbs, as per Ruled.me. The USDA reports that a serving of pinot noir has around four grams of carbs, and 1.5-ounce pour of bourbon in diet cola has short of what one carb, as indicated by Nutritionix. You can likewise swap out tonic for soft drink in blended beverages for an additional decrease in net carbs. Be set up for more regrettable aftereffects on the off chance that you drink while following a keto diet.

Eating a carb-overwhelming feast before drinking can shield you from getting alcoholic too rapidly. By a similar token, after an exacting keto diet can prompt turning out to be inebriated all the more rapidly and enduring a more awful aftereffect.

Coconut

There's a wealth of coconut items available, from coconut water and coconut flour to coconut oil. Coconut cream has for quite some time been a staple fixing in Asian foods and is utilized to plan rich and delightful dishes, for example, Thai curry and chicken tikka masala.

Coconut cream is made by bubbling coconut substance with water. Despite the fact that it's arranged a similar path as coconut milk, it has a more extravagant and thicker consistency. It's an ideal expansion for your keto dishes when you're searching for a rich and extraordinary flavor.

Coconut water is the liquid found inside new coconuts. This normally sweet water contains 45 calories for each serving and is stacked with potassium and different electrolytes, making it an ideal swap for sugary, added substance loaded games drinks. Coconut meat alludes to the white, palatable bit of the coconut. It very well may be eaten crude, cooked, or transformed into an assortment of other coconut items, for example, oil, milk, and cream. Coconut milk alludes to two totally different kinds of items. Genuine unsweetened coconut milk is made by taking equivalent pieces of destroyed coconut and water, and heating them to the point of boiling. The blend is then filtered through a cheesecloth and squeezed to discharge however much liquid as could reasonably be expected. Full-fat coconut milk is frequently sold in jars and has a consistency like entire cow's milk. The name coconut milk likewise normally alludes to the dairy milk substitute found on the racks of markets and wellbeing shops. This item is made after a similar procedure as above, however the destroyed coconut parts are additionally weakened and sustained to fulfill the national guidelines for a dairy milk substitution. This lighter form of coconut milk is commonly sold in containers and is far more slender than the unsweetened rendition. Make certain to peruse the fixing name as it could contain undesirable sugar, nourishment added substances, and stabilizers. You presently think about the most famous coconut subsidiaries and have the solution to your inquiry, "What is coconut cream?" Even better, you can make your own coconut cream in only a couple of simple advances.

Fermented Foods

There's a huge assortment of matured nourishment and beverages. The explanation we expend them is regularly in light of the fact that they're referred to for having amazing microorganisms, for example, probiotics and other great microscopic organisms.

These sorts of microscopic organisms have been connected to advancing a sound gut. Studies recommend that they have the capacities to help in weight reduction, support a strong safe framework, and improve assimilation. We'll investigate what the top-matured nourishments are on a keto diet and why precisely they're so useful for your wellbeing. To start, allows first investigate what continues during the aging procedure. Aging has been a piece of our way of life for a huge number of years and still lives on today. Be that as it may, what does maturing something really include?

Aging, basically, is a procedure that comprises of both yeast and different microorganisms separating the carbs in what you're attempting to age. It at that point gets transformed into the fundamental liquor and acids required to age and safeguard the blend. It's during this procedure that the probiotics and other microscopic organisms are made, which can yield a lot of medical advantages.

Salt

One of the trickier parts of the Ketogenic diet, particularly to beginners, comprehends the significance of expanding salt utilization. As our body advances from being a sugar burner to a fat terminator, it decreases the measure of sodium put away in the body along these lines requiring progressively salt in our eating routine. Since keto prohibits most helpful prepared nourishments that are high in sodium, the measure of sodium expended is normally diminished too. Therefore, sodium levels frequently drop causing unsavory reactions that can be effortlessly stayed away from. In the event that the entirety of this is different to you and simply beginning after a keto diet, this Guide to Getting Started on Keto is a phenomenal asset that is anything but difficult to follow.

The Role of salt in the Body

Sodium is a fundamental mineral that our body needs to direct water maintenance and parity water in and around cells. Without the best possible measure of sodium, we may encounter a large group of confusions, for example, anxiety, cerebrum mist, weakness, muscle cramps, belly inconveniences, and that's just the beginning. Sodium admission is considerably progressively significant while following a ketogenic diet since the sodium levels are lower than expected. Sodium and potassium cooperate so when the degree of sodium drops it legitimately influences potassium, which can exacerbate you feel.

1. Low Sodium Levels can Lead to "Keto Flu."

One of the less attractive impacts of the ketogenic diet is the "Keto Flu." This generally occurs inside the initial three to five days of following a keto diet. Indications incorporate inclination dormant, run-down, touchy, unmotivated, and so on. Our body doesn't approach the glucose it recently utilized for vitality and hasn't made the vital metabolic changes to effectively utilize fat for fuel yet.

Maybe the greatest reason for the keto influenza is parchedness and electrolyte unevenness. I as of late presented a straightforward guide on electrolytes on keto that streamline and clarifies electrolytes. Fortunately, the keto influenza is brief on low carb abstains from food. Remaining hydrated and adjusting your electrolytes is a straightforward procedure that can limit both the span and degree.

2. Low Sodium Levels can Lead to Tummy Troubles

An electrolyte awkwardness can prompt stomach related problems as your body needs sodium for the muscles in the stomach related tract to work appropriately. Many experience belly inconveniences, for example, stoppage and queasiness when sodium levels are out of equalization. In the event that you experience this, think about eating progressively salt, taking a magnesium supplement, or absorbing an Epsom Salt shower.

3. Low Electrolyte Levels Can Increase the Risk for Muscle Cramps

Muscle cramps, particularly around evening time, ordinarily show either gentle lack of hydration or low electrolyte levels, or both. This can be an extremely regular issue, particularly in the good 'ol days when beginning a ketogenic diet. Simple fixes for this incorporate drinking a sans sugar electrolyte drink like Ultima Replenisher or Powerade Zero (in the event that you follow a progressively apathetic keto diet), drinking water, taking the suitable enhancements to adjust electrolytes, and including increasingly salt keto in your eating routine.

- Pink Himalayan Salt (likewise called pink salt) – Is stacked with minerals like potassium, magnesium, and calcium to give some examples. It's a most loved decision among numerous on keto as it is progressively normal in structure and less prepared.

- Ocean Salt Sea salt is gotten from dissipated ocean water. With bigger precious stones, it is a lot saltier than ordinary table salt and furthermore contains included minerals.

Adjustments for special diet

The Modified Ketogenic Diet is a less prohibitive adaptation of great Keto, and can be useful when beginning the eating routine, or when decreasing down to a less prohibitive, long haul diet. Conveying a macronutrient proportion between 2:1 - 1:1, the eating regimen is planned in light of adaptability to expand consistence and lessening potential stomach related uneasiness and supplement insufficiency that can happen with long haul exemplary keto eating.

Fats to love, fats to hate

These sound fats are keto-accommodating yet advantage a wide range of eaters, as well. They're going to turn into your new BFFs.

Full-Fat Greek Yogurt

"Plain, full-fat Greek yogurt is a decent keto decision," says Julie Upton, R.D., fellow benefactor of Appetite for Health. "While it's high in protein, it's additionally high in immersed fats," she calls attention to. A blend of soaked and unsaturated fats is commonplace when following a keto supper plan, yet specialists despite everything concur that greasy nourishments wealthy in the immersed kind ought to be eaten in relative balance. "In any case, there are a few investigations that propose the immersed fat in dairy nourishments may not be as negative to heart wellbeing contrasted with soaked fats from meats and different sources," says Upton.

Macadamia Nuts

Nuts are certainly extraordinary compared to other solid fats to eat, however "not all nuts are made equivalent with regards to the keto diet," says Kasper. "For instance, cashews are higher in sugars. Macadamia nuts are an incredible fit since they are high in sound fat and low in carbs."

Virgin Coconut Oil

"Virgin coconut oil is a profoundly immersed fat, however it likewise gives some medium-chain triglycerides that are promptly scorched as fuel," says Upton. "One tablespoon of coconut oil has 117 calories and 14 grams of absolute fat, 12 of which are soaked. Utilizing virgin coconut oil will help guarantee that the oil contains a portion of the characteristic plant synthetics that may have other medical advantages." Still, Upton alerts that since coconut oil is so high in immersed fat, just utilize the greasy nourishment in limited quantities.

Salmon and Tuna

Look no farther than the ocean for sound fats to eat whether or not you're on the keto diet or not. "Greasy fish are keto-accommodating nourishment decisions since they give top notch protein and are wealthy in valuable omega-3 unsaturated fats, which help temper irritation and decrease the hazard for some ceaseless maladies."

Pumpkin Seeds

Seeds are another case of sound fats you'll need to eat on the reg—not simply around Halloween. "Seeds are supplement thick, high in mono and polyunsaturated unsaturated fats, and offer a healthy portion of protein," says Kasper. Truth be told, 75 percent of the fat in pumpkin seeds is monounsaturated or polyunsaturated.

One of the most beneficial greasy nourishments, these seeds likewise give fiber, protein, and different nutrients and minerals. "Pumpkin seeds are an incredible decision since they are plentiful in numerous minerals, for example, zinc, which underpins invulnerability, and magnesium, which is a mitigating."

Green growth

"Green growth is an uncelebrated yet truly great individual in the keto diet world," says Kasper. "With a lot of omega-3s (where did you think the fish get it?), in excess of 40 nutrients and minerals, and zero net carbs, green growth is a fantasy nourishment for the wellbeing cognizant keto weight watcher." It's not just about greasy nourishments—greasy beverages can help keep you in ketosis, as well. Toss a scoop of spirulina or chlorella, two sorts of green super powders produced using green growth, into your smoothie, or get the solid fat in tablet structure to take as an enhancement.

Olive Oil

Quality wellsprings of this sound fats to eat matter, so ensure you get the great stuff. "Excellent, cold-squeezed olive oil is delightful, high in monounsaturated unsaturated fats, and may have calming properties," says Danielle Aberman, R.D.N., a dietitian and co-proprietor of Migraine Relief Coach. "Diets high in olive oil have been appeared to bring down the danger of a few maladies."

To bring down generally speaking soaked fat admission while expending an eating routine with numerous greasy nourishments, utilize olive oil instead of spread to sauté vegetables and proteins. Furthermore, discard the locally acquired serving of mixed greens dressings and have a go at making your own straightforward vinaigrette utilizing olive oil, balsamic vinegar, and Dijon mustard.

Avocados

You most likely could have speculated avocado would be on the keto nourishments list since they're one of the least demanding and most delectable approaches to up your solid fat admission. "Avocados are wealthy in sound mono-and polyunsaturated fats, in addition to fiber and cancer prevention agents," says Upton. "Avocados are an extraordinary decision as a fat on the grounds that different fats, similar to oils, don't have the fiber of avocados." truth be told, the fiber content right now may assist you with feeling more full more, she says, which is constantly a success. This organic product additionally contributes cancer prevention agents and about 20 unique nutrients and minerals. ICYMI or have cut yourself awfully commonly here's the way to appropriately cut an avocado.

Eggs

Eggs are likewise a standout amongst other keto nourishments. "An enormous egg gives 13 basic supplements, 6 grams of the most great protein accessible, 5 grams of absolute fat, and 1.5 grams of immersed fat," says Upton. Furthermore, it's not simply the fat substance that makes them so astounding. "Eggs are likewise one of only a handful hardly any normal wellsprings of nutrient D, and they contain choline, which is fundamental for cerebrum wellbeing. They likewise have cell reinforcements that are useful for eye wellbeing.

Fats to hate
Despite the fact that fat makes up most of the calories on a ketogenic diet, not all wellsprings of fat are useful for your wellbeing, regardless of whether they fit into the macronutrient conveyance of your eating regimen plan.

Counterfeit trans fats

Falsely delivered trans fats are known for essentially expanding coronary illness hazard and ought to be maintained a strategic distance from, paying little mind to the kind of diet you're following. Trans fats are much of the time found in profoundly refined oils and monetarily arranged handled nourishments, for example, cakes, treats, baked goods, bread rolls, wafers, and other ultra-prepared tidbits. Trans fats might be shown on a fixing name under the names "mostly hydrogenated oils" or "shortening." It's ideal to keep away from nourishments that contain these fixings however much as could be expected.

Prepared meats

Prepared meats, for example, shop meat, hotdogs, salami, sausages, and relieved and smoked meats, are much of the time publicized as keto agreeable. While these nourishments actually fit into a ketogenic diet plan, a few investigations have discovered a relationship between high admission of handled meats and an expanded danger of malignancies of the stomach related tract.

In this way, it's ideal to keep your admission of these nourishments negligible. Rather, center around eating entire, insignificantly prepared nourishments however much as could be expected.

Seared nourishments

Pan fried nourishments are remembered for some ketogenic diet plans, however you might need to reconsider before adding them to yours. Singed nourishments will in general be high in trans-fats, which can expand your danger of coronary illness.

Particular kinds of profoundly refined oils commonly utilized for browning, for example, corn oil, frequently contain modest quantities of trans-fats. As the oils are warmed to high temperatures, more trans fats might be created.

Seared nourishment assimilates a lot of these fats, and successive utilization could prompt inconvenient wellbeing impacts after some time. Along these lines, downplay your admission of seared nourishments to help your wellbeing while at the same time following a ketogenic diet. The ketogenic diet is revolved around high-fat nourishments, yet a few wellsprings of fat are more advantageous than others. Greasy fish, avocados, coconut, olives, nuts, and seeds are a couple of instances of nutritious wellsprings of sound fats. To best help your wellbeing on the keto diet, pick fats from supplement thick, entire nourishments and evade those that originate from ultra-prepared oils, meats, and seared food sources.

Using keto fats and oil

With regards to adjusting to an eating regimen dependent on fats, it is imperative to comprehend that not all fats are made equivalent. To procure the weight reduction and generally speaking body medical advantages of the keto diet, it is suggested that you eat the correct sorts of fats not engineered trans fats from prepared nourishments, yet a moderate measure of immersed fats and an essential admission of polyunsaturated and monounsaturated fats. While meats, fish, nuts, regular dairy, and eggs are incredible wellsprings of the sort of fats you have to consolidate, perhaps the most ideal approaches to enhance your every day unsaturated fat admission is by utilizing cooking oils that are keto-accommodating at whatever point you make a home-prepared dinner.

The monounsaturated and polyunsaturated fats of characteristic, sound oils can help decrease your pulse, dispose of tummy fat, battle aggravation, lower cholesterol levels and increment heart wellbeing in any eating regimen. Joined with the nourishing impacts of different nourishments you eat on the keto diet, they will help add to the fruitful weight reduction and better wellbeing you are seeking after. Following are six of the best oils in any case when cooking for the keto diet.

1. Sesame Oil

Heart-sound, all-characteristic and pressed with a solid measurements of fundamental unsaturated fats, sesame oil is a seed oil with a rich, smooth flavor, and a nutty smell. This oil has a medium-high smoke point, which means it can arrive at generally high temperatures before starting to consume and smoke. At the point when oil begins to consume at its smoke point, the supplements in the oil are corrupting. It is critical to focus on the smoke point and legitimate use of every sort of oil to ensure you are not just getting the correct supplements from both your oil and your nourishment yet in addition keeping away from the irritation corrupted oils can trigger inside the body.

Utilize nutritious sesame oil to saute or fry your keto-accommodating nourishments, or add it to sauces and dressings you eat with your feast for a stunningly better stockpile of sound fats and supplements.

2. Avocado Oil

High in both monounsaturated fats and cancer prevention agents, avocado oil is a mellow, adaptable vegetable oil with an extra sound portion of nutrients An, E and D, just as proteins and potassium. In addition to the fact that this oils convey a healthy measure of unsaturated fats advantageous to your keto diet, however it additionally improves supplement retention and advances better cholesterol levels. With a staggeringly high smoke point, avocado oil is perfect for cooking in practically any style, including browning, barbecuing, broiling, sauteing, and burning. You can likewise utilize it for cold cooking purposes like marinades, dressings or plunges.

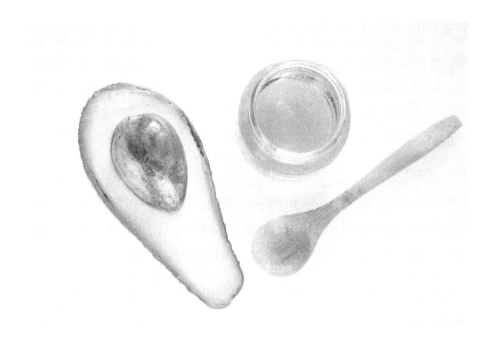

3. Coconut Oil

Extricated from the product of coconut palm trees, coconut oil is a keto-accommodating cooking oil high in soaked fat and of a comparable consistency to spread. Its medium-tie triglycerides assist speed with increasing the digestion and incite ketosis in moderate dosages. Coconut oil likewise has a generally high smoke point, making it perfect for sauteing, fricasseeing, cooking, and preparing keto nourishments as a substitute for spread.

4. Additional Virgin Olive Oil

With a low smoke point and an extraordinarily solid measure of monounsaturated fats and cell reinforcements, additional virgin olive oil is a chilly squeezed, grungy oil that holds a significant part of the flavor and supplements of the olives from which it is separated. In addition to the fact that this is virgin oil high in solid fats to agree to your keto diet, however it is likewise mind boggling, vigorous, rich and delightful, including notes of fruity, rich, and verdant flavors to your keto cooking manifestations.

Additional virgin olive oil has a low smoke point, be that as it may, so do whatever it takes not to utilize it for high-heat cooking or searing. Rather, join it in your dressings, marinades, and keto-accommodating tidbits. It additionally tastes flavorful with eggs, meats, and vegetables.

5. Hazelnut Oil

Solid in flavor and high in basic unsaturated fats to help your keto diet, hazelnut oil is a delightful, more extravagant option in contrast to olive oil. Cooked hazelnut oil is incredibly delightful and adds another layer of taste to any dish you join it into. Use hazelnut oil in your keto-accommodating preparing attempts, as a sound, greasy flavor substitute for pecans and pine nuts in natively constructed pesto, or as a scrumptious marinade, plate of mixed greens dressing or sauce.

PART TWO

Chapter Four: INTERNITTENT FASTING

What is Intermitent Fasting?

IF isn't an eating routine, it's a way of eating. It's a method for booking your dinners so you benefit from them. It doesn't change what you eat, it changes when you eat. It's an extraordinary method to get lean without going on an insane eating regimen or chopping your calories down to nothing. Indeed, more often than not you'll attempt to keep your calories a similar when you start discontinuous fasting. (The vast majority eat greater suppers during a shorter time allotment.) Additionally, it is a decent method to keep bulk on while getting lean. With all that stated the major reason individual's attempt this kind of fasting is to lose fat. Maybe in particular, irregular fasting is perhaps the least complex procedure we have for dropping terrible weight while keeping great load on in light of the fact that it requires almost no conduct change. This is an excellent thing since it implies discontinuous fasting falls into the class of "basic enough that you'll really do it, however significant enough that it will really have any kind of effect."

How does IF works?

To see how IF prompts fat misfortune we first need to comprehend the distinction between the fed state and the fasted state. Your body is in the fed state when it is processing and retaining nourishment. Regularly, the fed state begins when you start eating and goes on for three to five hours as your body processes and retains the nourishment you just ate. At the point when you are in the fed express, it's exceptionally difficult for your body to consume fat on the grounds that your insulin levels are high. After that timespan, your body goes into what is known as the post absorptive state, which is only an extravagant method for saying that your body isn't handling a feast. The post absorptive state goes on until 8 to 12 hours after your last supper, which is the point at which you enter the fasted state. It is a lot simpler for your body to consume fat in the fasted state in light of the fact that your insulin levels are low. At the point when you're in the fasted express your body can consume fat that has been out of reach during the fed state. Since we don't enter the fasted state until 12 hours after our last supper, it's uncommon that our bodies are right now state. This is one reason why numerous individuals who start discontinuous fasting will lose fat without changing what they eat, the amount they eat, or how regularly they work out. Fasting places your body in a fat consuming state that you once in a while make it to do, during a typical eating plan.

Why does IF works?

While IF might be a mainstream pattern in the eating regimen world nowadays, those attempting to get thinner or improve their general wellbeing should realize that it tends to be a hard arrangement to stick to. The methodology shifts back and forth between times of fasting and non-fasting during a specific timeframe. IF isn't about hardship, however about separating your calories uniquely in contrast to the three-full dinners daily in addition to a nibble routine. The explanation IF is believed to be successful in weight reduction is on the grounds that it expands your body's responsiveness to insulin. Insulin, a hormone that is discharged when you eat nourishment, causes your liver, muscle and fat cells to store glucose. In a fasting state, blood glucose levels drop, which prompts a lessening in insulin creation, flagging your body to begin consuming put away vitality (starches). Following 12 hours of fasting, your body comes up short on put away vitality and starts consuming put away fat.

What effects does it have on your body Hormones?

The advantages of IF are buzzing in the wellbeing scene with inquire about supporting its capacity to decrease inflammation, heal the gut, and increment cell fix. As a functional medication practitioner it's a restorative device that I suggest all the time for a large number of my patients. While restricting nourishment admission for a while can do ponders for your wellbeing, there are a few concerns in regards to the potential symptoms it could have on hormonal wellbeing, particularly for those with thyroid issues, adrenal weakness or other hormone uneven characters. So how about we jump profound into the hormone-fasting association with assistance decide whether this could be a decent mending device for you:

1. Fat putting away and hunger hormones: (leptin, insulin, + ghrelin)

Discontinuous fasting becomes the overwhelming focus in its job in improving yearning, digestion, and glucose influencing hormones. At the point when patients come in with blood sugar problems I like to prescribe IF because of its demonstrated capacity to increase metabolism and lower insulin obstruction. In the event that you have a glucose issue and need to have a go at fasting it's vital to work with your primary care physician who can screen you and easing back increment your length of fasting as your glucose stabilizes. Leptin opposition, another hormonal obstruction design which prompts weight put on and weight reduction obstruction, has likewise been appeared to improve with IF.

What's more, in the event that you figure fasting would make you increasingly eager, reconsider. Irregular fasting has been appeared to emphatically influence the craving hormone ghrelin which can directly improve brain dopamine levels. This is the ideal case of the truth of the gut-mind pivot association.

2. Estrogen and progesterone

Your cerebrum and ovaries impart through the mind ovary hub or hypothalamic-pituitary-gonadal (HPG) pivot. Your cerebrum discharges hormones to your ovaries to flag them to discharge estrogen and progesterone. In the event that your HPG hub isn't functioning admirably it can influence your general wellbeing and lead to issues with richness. With regards to IF, ladies are generally more delicate than men. This is because of the way that ladies have more kiss peptin, which makes more noteworthy affectability to fasting. If not done appropriately, IF can make ladies mess up their cycle and lose their hormones. While more research should be done it would bode well to legitimately reason that this hormonal move could influence digestion and richness as well.

Presently this to state since each individual is unique, this doesn't mean you can never attempt intermittent fasting. You may simply need to go at it with an alternate methodology. This fasting can be an incredible method to systematically bring fasting into your daily schedule.

3. Adrenal hormones (cortisol):

Cortisol is your body's fundamental pressure hormone and is discharged by your adrenal organs which sit directly on your kidneys. At the point when your mind adrenal (HPA) hub is lost it can prompt awkwardness in cortisol. This high and low rollercoaster winds up driving to adrenal weakness. I've discovered that individuals with dysfunctions with their circadian beat don't deal with discontinuous fasting great. Nonetheless, attempting a moderate novice irregular fasting convention or the crescendo fasting could approve of somebody checking your advancement.

4. Thyroid hormones:

Your thyroid is sovereign of all hormones influencing each and every cell in your body. No other hormone has that power. On the off chance that your thyroid hormones are not working ideally, at that point nothing is. There are a wide range of types of thyroid problems all of which can be affected diversely by irregular fasting. Along these lines, I suggest working with a useful medication professional who can work with your particular wellbeing case.

In the event that you presume that you may have a hormone issue look at my guide on the theme to find some more solutions to your waiting inquiries. On the off chance that you realize you are obvious to begin look no further to begin your irregular fasting venture:

Beginners:

The 8-6 window plan: One simple way to IF is to just eat between 8 am and 6pm. This allows for a long fasting period within a reasonable timeframe.

The 12-6 window plan: I personally do this plan during my workweek. This is the same as the last plan but extends the fast a couple more hours into lunchtime. I fill my morning with big cups of water and antioxidant-rich matcha tea.

Intermediate:

Modified 2-day plan: Eat clean for five days and then restrict calorie intake to 700 on any two other days. Limited calorie intake can have similar effects as full fasting.

The 5-2 plan: Eat clean for five days and fully fast for two nonconsecutive days a week.

Advanced:

Every-other-day plan: Fast fully every other day. While intense, it can be very effective for some people.

Nutrition for women over 60 and hormonal problems

Want a simple recipe to fight aging? The ingredients are easy to find. The right mix of nutrients -- and some regular exercise will let you feel and look your best.

When you eat right, you'll help get your weight under control, keep your bones strong, and prevent heart disease. It's all about making smart choices.

Nutrition Basics

Boost calcium and vitamin D. That means three to four 8-ounce servings of low-fat dairy every day. If you are lactose-intolerant, eat hard cheese, yogurt, or kefir; canned salmon; broccoli; and legumes. You can also try food or drinks, like orange juice, that have the nutrients added in by the manufacturer. They'll say "fortified" on the label.

If your doctor says you don't get enough calcium in your diet, he may suggest you take supplements that have 1,000 to 1,600 milligrams of the nutrient.

Eat more fruits, veggies, whole grains, and legumes. These will give you plenty of disease-fighting antioxidants. Focus on variety every day, including vegetables with different colors.

Get enough fiber. You don't have to look far. Some good sources are:

Legumes

Whole wheat pasta

Whole-grain cereals and breads

Oatmeal

Brown rice

Popcorn

Fresh fruits and veggies

Take a daily multivitamin. It will fill any gaps in your nutrition picture. But make sure it's tailored for your age group. When you're over 60, you need less iron than younger women.

Eat lean proteins. Try foods such as skinless chicken, fatty fish like salmon (with omega-3 fats), and vegetable protein, including soy.

Enjoy a vegetarian meal a few times a week. Plant-based diets have lots of advantages. They're low in calories but rich in vitamins, minerals, and antioxidants.

Cut down on salt. Too much salt is linked to high blood pressure. The recently-published 2015 Dietary Guidelines once again remind everyone to limit salt to 2,300 milligrams a day.

Choose fats wisely. Avoid trans and saturated fats. They're often hidden in things like:

Butter

Stick margarine

Processed foods

Desserts

Doughnuts

"Good fats" can be found in olive oil, and some, but not all, vegetable oils like canola, as well as food like:

Nuts and seeds

Avocado

Cold-water fish such as salmon and tuna

Curb the sweets. Limit sugary drinks and deserts and sweetened dairy products. They can be loaded with calories and have little nutrition.

What to eat while intermittent fasting for women over 60

There are no specifications or restrictions about what type or how much food to eat while following intermittent fasting. People embarking on IF should eat a well-balanced diet is the key to losing weight, maintaining energy levels, and sticking with the diet. Anyone attempting to lose weight should focus on nutrient-dense foods, like fruits, veggies, whole grains, nuts, beans, seeds, as well as dairy and lean proteins. In other words, eat plenty of the below foods and you won't end up in a hangry rage while fasting. Th list of food to eat while intermittent fasting includes:

1. Water

2. Avocado

3. Fish

4. Cruciferous Veggies

5. Potatoes

5. Beans and Legumes

6. Probiotics

7. Berries

8. Eggs

9. Nuts

10. Whole Grains

How intermittent fasting affects women at this age?

While some nutrition experts contend that IF only works because it helps people naturally limit food intake, others disagree. They believe that intermittent fasting results are better than typical meal schedules with the same amount of calories and other nutrients. Studies have even suggested that abstaining from food for several hours a day does more than just limit the amount of calories you consume. These are some metabolic changes that IF causes that might help account for synergistic benefits:

Insulin: During the fasting period, lower insulin levels will help improve fat burning.

HGH: While insulin levels drop, HGH levels rise to encourage fat burning and muscle growth.

Noradrenaline: In response to an empty belly, the nervous system will send this chemical to cells to let them know they need to release fat for fuel.

Is Intermittent Fasting Healthy?

Is intermittent fasting safe? Remember that you're only supposed to fast for twelve to sixteen hours and not for days at a time. You've still got plenty of time to enjoy a satisfying and healthy diet. Of course, some older women may need to eat frequently because of metabolic disorders or the instructions on prescriptions. In that case, you should discuss your eating habits with your medical provider before making any changes.

While it's not technically fasting, some doctors have reported intermittent fasting benefits by allowing such easy-to-digest food as whole fruit during the fasting window." was a popular weight loss book that suggested eating only fruit after supper and before lunch.

Chapter Five: Intermittent fasting and types

IF can be utilized as meager or as regularly to suit your necessities. You may even prefer to blend and match consistently, rehearsing some every day, and others month to month or yearly. The sum total of what strategies has been demonstrated to be viable, yet through research, experimentation, you will locate the one that suits you best.

16:8 method

The 16:8 is one of the most famous types of discontinuous fasting that can be handily consolidated into every day life. Basically, you confine eating to an eight hour window with 2–3 dinners, and quick for 16 hours.

For instance, quit having after supper at 6pm, and draw out breakfast till 10am the next day, eat for 8 hours, and the cycle starts once more. You can change the planning as per your calendar maybe you like to eat prior or later in the day. This sort of fasting is entirely sensible and suggested for the vast majority

14:10 method

In contrast to the mainstream 16:8 strategy, it has another proportion of fasting and taking care of periods. Discontinuous fasting 14:10 has an eating window of 10 hours and fasting window of 14 hours. One regular way to deal with doing this is to eat ordinarily in the hours between 9 a.m. what's more, 7 p.m. The period between 7 p.m. also, 9 a.m. the following day is the fasting window. During the taking care of period, you can eat your typical dinners and tidbits. In like manner, during the fasting window, you are not permitted to eat any calories. Be that as it may, you can drink water and unsweetened espresso or green tea.

20:4 method

The 20:4 is a kind of time prohibitive eating dependent on a 20 hour quick, with a four hour eating window. By and large, you can eat however much you might want during the four hour devouring, yet of course, it is hard to expend an excessive number of calories during such a brief timeframe outline.

The four hour eating window commonly occurs at night, however can be any piece of the day that suits you. For instance, you can eat two dinners somewhere in the range of 2pm and 6pm, and quick for the staying 20 hours.

This would be appropriate for the individuals who are sure with discontinuous fasting, are occupied day laborers and don't have the opportunity to eat, don't feel hungry during the day, or find that eating makes them less profitable and languid.

20:4 can likewise be utilized for those uncommon events whether you're taking off for a night dinner, or going to devour a tasty, feast with loved ones

The warrior method

The warrior diet includes fasting for 20 hours medium-term and during the day, and afterward indulging during a four-hour window at night. This standard depends on the possibility that our crude precursors went through their days chasing and assembling and would eat around evening time.

12:12 strategy

The key is to go fasting for 24 hours between every dinner. For instance, eat at 7pm on the very first moment and quick till 7pm the following day. Then again you can decide to eat prior (for breakfast or lunch), and quick for 24 hours till the following day. The thought is that you eat a dinner every day, except permit your body to quick for expanded periods. This sort of fasting is typically done a few times for each week, however can be received all the more often.

5:2 Method

The 5:2 or quick eating routine empowers fasting for 2 days of the week. For any two days, calories are limited to 600–600 for ladies and men, separately. Calories can be spread out over various suppers for the duration of the day, or eaten across the board. For the staying five days, eating isn't confined by fasting. For instance, you can eat ordinarily consistently, aside from Tuesday and Saturday, when you just eat 600–600 calories (2 dinners of 260 calories, or one feast of 600kcals) in the day.

Eat-stop-eat

This is one that I would suggest for any individual who is going back and forth about discontinuous fasting, or feels overpowered by setting prohibitive fasting times. This is a delicate prologue to irregular fasting, which is driven by your way of life and body. It is ideal for the individuals who don't care to feel confined, or get debilitated in the event that they don't meet the criteria of their eating routine. You essentially permit yourself to skip dinners in the event that you don't feel hungry, or too occupied to even think about eating.

Alternate day method

As the name recommends, this includes fasting each other day. On fasting days, eating is limited to one dinner of 600 calories, or complete fasting (without calories). Interchange days, you can eat ordinarily (similarly as with all fasting, nourishing ketosis is suggested for this time.) Long-term, this is a serious technique for fasting, and likely impractical. Regardless of what discontinuous fasting you choose to follow, recollect that calories and nourishment quality are still significant and shouldn't be ignored. Frequently individuals can side-line nourishment quality or over enjoy on calories as they utilize discontinuous fasting as a wellbeing net. Over the long haul, this won't be powerful and your wellbeing will be undermined.

Chapter Six: Approach to intermittent fasting

It very well may be trying to adhere to a discontinuous fasting program. The accompanying tips may assist individuals with been on target and foster the advantages of it:

Remaining hydrated: Drink heaps of water and without calorie drinks, for example, home grown teas, for the duration of the day.

Abstaining from fixating on nourishment: Plan a lot of interruptions on fasting days to abstain from contemplating nourishment, for example, making up for lost time with administrative work or heading out to see a film.

Resting and unwinding: Dodge strenuous exercises on fasting days, albeit light exercise such as yoga may be gainful.

Making the most of each calorie: In the event that the picked arrangement permits a few calories during fasting periods, select supplement thick nourishments that are wealthy in protein, fiber, and empowering fats. Models incorporate beans, lentils, eggs, fish, nuts, and avocado.

Eating high-volume nourishments: Select filling yet low-calorie nourishments, which incorporate popcorn, crude vegetables, and organic products with high water content, for example, grapes and melon.

Expanding the taste without the calories: Season dinners liberally with garlic, herbs, flavors, or vinegar. These nourishments are incredibly low in calories yet are brimming with season, which may assist with lessening sentiments of craving.

Picking supplement thick nourishments after the fasting time frame. Eating nourishments that are high in fiber, vitamins, minerals, and different supplements assists with keeping glucose levels consistent and forestall supplement lacks. A fair eating regimen will likewise add to weight reduction and generally speaking wellbeing.
There are a wide range of approaches to do IF, and there is no single arrangement that will work for everybody. People will encounter the best outcomes on the off chance that they evaluate the different styles to perceive what suits their way of life and inclinations.

Benefits of Intermittent fasting for women over 60

As we sail past 60, we will in general look out for things that will improve our experience in age, from serums and enhancements to diets, medications, and conventions. The items available are really perpetual, however incidentally, perhaps the best thing you can accomplish for your maturing body doesn't include purchasing or getting tied up with anything.

You may have known about irregular fasting, which includes reasonable, exchanging times of eating and not eating, otherwise known as fasting. The exploration is entirely evident that irregular fasting is gainful from numerous points of view, and this might be particularly valid for more seasoned grown-ups. The following are five advantages of irregular fasting, alongside how to do it:

1. It helps fix cellular forms in your body.

The cellular part is not all bad as we age, however fasting has been appeared to prompt your body's cell fix forms, improve hormone work, and even improves the capacity of qualities identified with sickness security and life span.

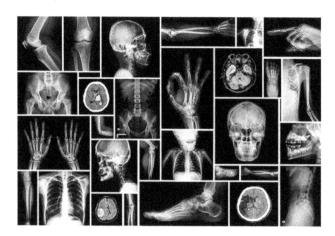

2. It advances weight reduction particularly gut fat.

Gut fat means that instinctive fat, which lies somewhere inside the stomach cavity, encompassing your organs and adding to infection. Losing gut fat is intense, particularly as we age, however as per an ongoing writing survey, discontinuous fasting can prompt lost four to seven percent of your abdomen outline.

An ongoing report found that discontinuous fasting can cause in general weight reduction of three to eight percent more than three to 24 weeks.

3. It helps lessens aggravation and oxidative pressure.

Irritation and oxidative pressure are significant supporters of ailment as we age, and they add to the unmistakable indications of maturing. This fasting decreases markers of oxidative pressure and irritation in overweight grown-ups.

4. It may help forestall Alzheimer's infection.

A huge collection of research shows that irregular fasting is useful for the mind, advancing the development of new nerve cells, shielding against cerebrum harm coming about because of stroke, and expanding levels of a hormone called cerebrum determined neurotrophic factor or BDNF.

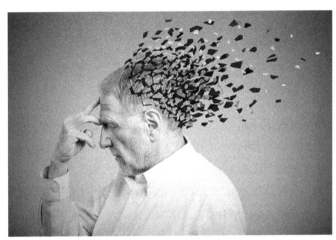

5. It may broaden your life.

A scope of ongoing examinations have additionally discovered that irregular fasting broadened the member's life expectancy. One examination found that rodents fasting each other day lived 83 percent longer than non-fasting rodents. Moreover, the pace of maturing was eased back in the fasting rodents, and their body weight and development rates were decreased.

Myths about intermittent fasting

Fasting has gotten progressively normal. Truth be told, IF, a dietary example that cycles between times of fasting and eating, is frequently advanced as a supernatural occurrence diet. However, not all things caught wind of feast recurrence and your wellbeing is valid. The following are myths about fasting and dinner recurrence.

1. Skipping breakfast makes you fat

One progressing fantasy is that morning meal is the most significant feast of the day.

Individuals normally accept that skipping breakfast prompts unnecessary yearning, desires, and weight gain. One 16-week study in 283 grown-ups with overweight and heftiness watched no weight distinction between the individuals who had breakfast and the individuals who didn't. Consequently, breakfast doesn't generally influence your weight, despite the fact that there might be some individual changeability. A few examinations even recommend that individuals who get thinner over the long haul will in general have breakfast. In addition, kids and young people who have breakfast will in general perform better at school. Thusly, it's imperative to focus on your specific needs. Breakfast is gainful for certain individuals, while others can skip it with no negative outcomes.

2. Eating much of the time supports your digestion

Numerous individuals accept that eating more dinners builds your metabolic rate, making your body consume more calories overall. Your body surely consumes a few calories processing suppers. This is named the thermic impact of nourishment. By and large, TEF utilizes around 10% of your complete calorie consumption. Nonetheless, what is important is the absolute number of calories you expend not what number of suppers you eat. Eating six 600-calorie dinners has a similar impact as eating three 1,000-calorie suppers. Given a normal TEF of 10%, you'll consume 300 calories in the two cases.

Various investigations exhibit that expanding or diminishing dinner recurrence doesn't influence complete calories consumed.

3. Eating much of the time diminishes hunger

A few people accept that occasional eating forestalls yearnings and exorbitant appetite. However, the proof is blended. Albeit a few investigations propose that eating increasingly visit dinners prompts decreased yearning, different examinations have discovered no impact or even expanded appetite levels.

One investigation that thought about eating three or six high-protein meals every day found that eating three dinners decreased yearning all the more successfully. All things considered, reactions may rely upon the person. In the event that regular eating lessens your yearnings, it's most likely a smart thought. All things considered, there's no proof that eating or eating more often reduces hunger for everybody. 4. Visit dinners can assist you with shedding pounds

Since eating all the more as often as possible doesn't support your digestion, it moreover doesn't have any impact on weight reduction. In reality, an examination in 16 grown-ups with stoutness thought about the impacts of eating 3 and 6 meals per day and found no distinction in weight, fat misfortune, or craving.

A few people guarantee that eating frequently makes it harder for them to hold fast to a healthy diet. Notwithstanding, on the off chance that you find that eating all the more frequently makes it simpler for you to eat less calories and less lousy nourishment, don't hesitate to stay with it.

4. Irregular fasting causes you to lose muscle

A few people accept that when you quick, your body begins consuming muscle for fuel. In spite of the fact that this occurs with eating less junk food when all is said in done, no proof recommends that it happens more with irregular fasting than different strategies. Then again, considers demonstrate that irregular fasting is better for keeping up bulk. Strikingly, irregular fasting is well known among many bodybuilders, who find that it keeps up muscle close by a low muscle to fat ratio.

5. Irregular fasting is awful for your wellbeing

While you may have heard bits of gossip that irregular fasting hurts your wellbeing, examines uncover that it has several impressive medical advantages. For instance, it changes your quality articulation identified with life span and resistance and has been appeared to draw out life expectancy in creatures.

It additionally has significant advantages for metabolic wellbeing, for example, improved insulin sensitivity and diminished oxidative pressure, irritation, and coronary illness chance. It might likewise support cerebrum wellbeing by raising degrees of mind inferred neurotrophic factor (BDNF), a hormone that may secure against melancholy and different other states of mind.

Various fantasies get propagated about intermittent fasting and feast recurrence. Be that as it may, a large number of these bits of gossip are not valid. For instance, eating littler, increasingly visit dinners doesn't support your digestion or assist you with shedding pounds. In addition, discontinuous fasting is a long way from undesirable and may offer various advantages. It's essential to counsel sources or do a little research before forming a hasty opinion about your metabolism and generally speaking wellbeing.

Intermittent fasting and Autophagy

Another enormous advantage connected to fasting is autophagy, which signifies "self-eating": it alludes to when the body eats up and reuses dead or harmed cells. Fasting has been connected to expanded autophagy, particularly in the mind, which may be the reason it's occasionally connected to bring down dangers of some neurodegenerative ailments.

Once more, there's very little data here, however a recent report on mice found that guys experience altogether more autophagy in the cerebrum when fasting than females. Be that as it may, on the other hand, those are mice. Set forth plainly, there's right now not even close to enough proof to make the case that human guys and females experience various degrees of autophagy.

What eat and don't eat during IF

One slip-up that novices regularly make is eating everything without exception during all their eatings window. They incorrectly accept that all calories are equivalent and that their body will consume what they eat during the following fasting stage. The body, obviously, consumes calories, and particularly fat, during your quick, yet for the best outcomes, you should even now mind your eating regimen.

A few nourishments to abstain from during discontinuous fasting:

- Quick Foods

- Prepared Foods

- Desserts

- Basic Carbs

- Sugary Sodas

- Improved Fruit Juice

- Solid Foods to Enjoy During Your Eating Window

Calories despite everything tally, and you ought to get the most sustenance conceivable from each calorie you eat. In a perfect world, you ought to eat similar sorts of sound nourishments during IF that you would eat on any solid eating regimen. That implies eating loads of vegetables, lean protein, sound fats, fish, entire grains, dairy, and vegetables. While these nutritional categories hold the way in to your irregular fasting achievement, a few decisions are still superior to other people.

Veggies incorporate a great deal of cruciferous veggies, for example, broccoli, cauliflower, and brussel grows into your eating regimen. They have more fiber to help in absorption, and they likewise assist you with feeling more full.

Beans and Legumes: Black beans, chickpeas, and peas are useful for expanding your vitality as well as a decent wellspring of protein.

Organic products and Berries: You need to abstain from over-burdening on organic product since they contain a ton of normal sugar that meddles with insulin levels. Berries are a superior decision due to the high supplement and cancer prevention agent content. Adding berries and nuts to plates of mixed greens will assist you with getting a decent variety of sustenance in a solitary tasty serving.

Nuts: Nuts contain great fat and a ton of cancer prevention agents. Albeit nutritious, they are additionally high in calories. Almonds, pecans, hazelnuts, cashews are an incredible decision.

Protein Lean meat, chicken, and fish are altogether acceptable wellsprings of protein. Eggs are another acceptable source and they are quick and simple to get ready. Eating more protein fulfills your craving longer. It additionally encourages you manufacture muscle that is expected to support your digestion.

Fish Seafood is stuffed with supplements, particularly omega-3 unsaturated fats. Individuals who ordinarily eat more Omega-3 diminish their danger of coronary illness, dementia, and despondency. Salmon, shrimp, and trout are some ideal supplement thick decisions.

Entire Grains: Whole grains are another acceptable protein source that is additionally wealthy in fiber. For rice and bread – pick entire grain ones. Additionally, attempt some new nourishments like sorghum, spelt, or kamut, and perhaps you'll discover something that accommodates your taste and your new eating style.

Sound Fats: Nuts and fish are acceptable wellsprings of solid fats. When choosing fats for cooking, olive oil and coconut oil are your best decisions.

Dairy: You may be enticed to eat low-fat dairy, yet it isn't the best decision. Low-fat dairy items frequently likewise have fewer supplements.

Drinks to have and avoid while IF

It's most likely nothing unexpected that you ought to drink plenty of water to keep you hydrated during the two periods of fasting. Be that as it may, you aren't constrained to drinking water. You can likewise have zero-calorie beverages during both the fasting and eating window. Notwithstanding, fake sugars in diet soft drinks can trigger sugar yearnings. Another extraordinary choice is bone broth. Bone soup is famous for its amazingly high dietary benefit and furthermore assists with battling nourishment yearnings. There aren't any unbreakable guidelines on what to eat during irregular fasting. The most significant thing is to stay with the calendar and eat as sound as could be allowed. On the off chance that you diminish the quantity of calories you eat and settle on progressively nutritious decisions, you can rely on getting in shape and feeling much improved.

Intermittent fasting (IF) is an example of fasting and eating over a characterized timespan. There are numerous different types of fasting that you can do to suit your way of life.

There are two sections to IF: taking care of window (eating) and fasting window (not eating). On the off chance that isn't characterized by specific nourishments, yet we generally recommend low carb during times of eating.

By definition, fasting is the point at which you cease from eating or drinking any calories. Numerous individuals use fasting for explicit wellbeing benefits autophagy (cell turnover), ketosis, fat consuming and insulin affectability. Notwithstanding what you may think, fasting isn't about drying out and starvation. There are sure beverages and nourishment you can expend that impersonate the fasted state, and permit related advantages to happen.

The following is a gone through of 8 unique nourishments and beverages you can devour during a quick to assist you with arriving at your wellbeing objectives.

Water

Plain water is perhaps the best choice to drink during a quick. It will keep you hydrated and doesn't have an enzymic impact. For the fasting perfectionists, anything that causes an enzymic impact will break a quick for more data, look at Dr. Ronda Patrick. Water is likewise an extraordinary device for banishing cravings for food. It will top off your belly.

Stick to present or shining water. To include enhance, you can mix it with cuts of lemon, berries, cucumber or a cool tea implantations. It's essential to keep hydrated during a quick, so mean to drink between 1-3 liters of wa

Tea gives extraordinary solace and can be delighted in bounteous sums while you quick. Feeling colder than typical while fasting is ordinary. Tea will keep you warm and cause you to feel full, without the caffeine hit you ordinarily get from espresso.

Drink home grown, dark, oolong, green and white tea, without anything included. It would be ideal if you know that tannins in tea can cause queasiness on the off chance that you drink them on a vacant stomach. You may need to look around to discover one that concurs with you.

Coffe

Indeed, coffe is on the rundown unified moan of alleviation! Coffee is a compelling hunger suppressant and can be utilized as a feast swap for breakfast or lunch. Research has even demonstrated that espresso utilization can expand ketone creation and direct blood glucose, which improves metabolic wellbeing. In any case, a few people are especially delicate to caffeine and it can raise blood glucose levels tragically I'm one of those people, so I maintain a strategic distance from it.

Taking Coffee on an unfilled stomach can make you increasingly touchy to caffeine, so you may encounter heartburn, resentful stomach, and uneasiness, a bad case of nerves or restless evenings. In the event that you're gesturing along to this, at that point attempt to keep away from espresso or utilize swiss water decaffeinated espresso.

Drink dark espresso, without anything included, and limit utilization to prior in the day so it doesn't disturb your rest.

Apple Cider Vinegar

Apple juice vinegar is stacked with wellbeing properties — help solid gut microbiome, helps absorption, improves insulin affectability, brings down blood glucose and expands satiety. Apple juice vinegar is generally comprised of water, acidic corrosive and gut adoring probiotics. It has an exceptionally minor calorie content and won't break your quick.

Apple juice vinegar will help quiet yearnings and extinguish thirst. Weaken 1-2 tablespoons in still or shimmering water, and appreciate!

Bone Broth

Bone soup is a rich wellspring of minerals, and will help recharge electrolytes, which are typically lost during a quick. It is additionally an extraordinary wellspring of collagen, which will reestablish and fix the gut lining.

Bone juices contains protein, which can cause an insulin spike and break a quick. Notwithstanding, the calorie content is impressively low, so it will keep you in ketosis. Likewise with impenetrable espresso, if drinking bone stock implies that you draw out fasting, or think that its simpler, at that point I would state, move with that. It will assist you with fixing insulin affectability, which is a definitive objective! Utilize natively constructed bone stock just, to stay away from added substances and fillers. Here's a recipe!

Salt

Electrolyte misfortune is a typical and ordinary reaction during discontinuous fasting. Therefore, you may encounter dry mouth and thirst, in spite of your exertion of drinking gallons of water.

Salt is an extraordinary method to renew electrolytes, wash down the sense of taste and hose hunger. Utilize a little piece at once, a couple of touches on your tongue, and let it work its magic — in no time, appetite will evaporate, alongside that ghastly covering in the mouth.

Tips and Tricks for successful Intermitting fasting for women over 60
Sometimes it's difficult to adhere to a routine especially, Intermittent Fasting.

The following tips will surely assist individuals with been on target, focusing and utilizing the advantages of IF:

Remaining hydrated: Drink loads of water and without calorie drinks, for example, home grown teas, for the duration of the day.

Abstaining from fixating on nourishment: Plan a lot of interruptions on fasting days to abstain from contemplating nourishment, for example, getting up to speed with desk work or heading out to see a film.

Resting and unwinding: Evade strenuous exercises on fasting days, albeit light exercise such as yoga may be advantageous.

Making the most of each calorie: In the event that the picked arrangement permits a few calories during fasting periods, select supplement thick nourishments that are wealthy in protein, fiber, and invigorating fats: Models incorporate beans, lentils, eggs, fish, nuts, and avocado.

Eating high-volume nourishments. Select filling yet low-calorie nourishments, which incorporate popcorn, crude vegetables, and natural products with high water content, for example, grapes and melon.

Expanding the taste without the calories: Season dinners liberally with garlic, herbs, flavors, or vinegar. These nourishments are amazingly low in calories yet are brimming with enhance, which may assist with lessening sentiments of yearning.

Picking supplement thick nourishments after the fasting time frame: Eating nourishments that are high in fiber, vitamins, minerals, and different supplements assists with keeping glucose levels consistent and forestall supplement lacks. A reasonable eating routine will likewise add to weight reduction and by and large wellbeing.

Who can do Intermittent fasting and who cannot?

While intermittent fasting may be easy for some, it might not be that easy for other. However, the following will help you through the process, making it quite easy to do.

IF, isn't simply one more method for saying "free ride. Randomly skipping dinners while proceeding to eat an eating regimen high in prepared nourishments won't assist you with losing fat or improve your wellbeing. So while there's nobody "right" approach to work on fasting, any conventional convention will include a specific measure of consideration regarding healthful particulars. You must be set up to accomplish that work. Some will view IF as excessively badly arranged or inconvenient to rehearse. What's more, for other people, its dangers far exceed any potential advantages. Truth be told, for certain individuals IF could be absolute risky.

Before you avoid your next feast, you most likely need to know whether you fall into that class. Here's the lowdown, in light of various contextual analyses and a limited quantity of distributed research.

IF: Green Light

Everyone is can make the most of IF, when

- you have a past filled with observing calorie and nourishment admission (e.g., you've "abstained from food" previously)

- you're as of now an accomplished exerciser

- you're single or you don't have kids

- your accomplice (in the event that you have one) is incredibly steady

- your activity permits you to have times of low execution while you adjust to another arrangement

- you're a male

The initial five components will permit you to incorporate the conventions with your way of life all the more effectively, while the last condition (being male) appears to influence results.

IF: Yellow Light Meanwhile, on the chance that you meet the following criteria;

- You're hitched or have kids

- You have execution arranged or customer confronting employments

- You contend in sport/games

- You're female

Once more, the three major conditions make it a lot harder to follow IF conventions and may make it illogical for you. In addition, attempting to IF may strife with execution objectives for your game.

With respect to the last condition, some experimenters suggest that for ladies, fasting causes sleeplessness, uneasiness, sporadic periods, and different signs of hormone dysregulation.

In particular, women appear to charge worse on the stricter types of discontinuous fasting than men do. So in case you're female and you need to take a stab at fasting, I prescribe starting with a casual methodology.

IF: Red Light

At long last, there are a few people who truly shouldn't waste time with IF. Should in case you meet the following criteria, we advised not to embark on IF when

- You're pregnant

- You have a background marked by cluttered eating

- You are incessantly focused

- You don't rest well

- You're new to abstain from food and exercise

In case you're new to eat less carbs and exercise, irregular fasting may resemble an enchantment projectile for weight reduction. However, you'd be much more intelligent to address any dietary inadequacies before you begin trying different things with fasts. Guarantee you're beginning from a strong wholesome stage first.

Pregnant women have additional vitality needs, so in case you're beginning a family, this isn't an ideal opportunity to quick. Likewise on the off chance that you are under chronic stress and/or not dozing. Your body needs sustaining, not extra pressure.

Does IF have different effects on men and women?

No one is stating ladies are more sensitive than men. In any case, it's conceivable that irregular fasting influences people in an unexpected way. We could do with much more research right now no methods is this a sweeping speculation; a lot of men despise fasting and a lot of ladies blossom with it. All things considered, there is proof to recommend that ladies may be increasingly vulnerable to negative impacts, so we met a weight reduction centered doctor and took a gander at the exploration to address these issues.

The procedure is profoundly directed in ladies as it's engaged with ovulation, which is dependent on cycles and calendars. It's conceivable that among ladies, gonadotropin discharging hormone is all the more effortlessly upset by changes to one's propensities and routines, so skirting one's typical supper can some of the time cause more uneasiness among ladies than men. Ladies have been appeared to have a more significant level of protein called kisspeptin, which makes it more noteworthy to fasting. While more research is should have been done on this, it bodes well to coherently reason that the hormonal move (from fasting) can influence the digestion.

Can IF extend a women fertility?

Could fasting permit more established women to have kids? That is the ramifications of two new examinations which recommend that limiting nourishment may balance a portion of the loss of egg quality and amount that accompanies maturing. The discoveries may even empower new eggs to be made without any preparation.

It's not yet evident whether the discoveries stretch out to people, yet a superior comprehension of the instruments included may in the long run make it simpler for more established ladies to tolerate kids.

Starving worms

That is the place the subsequent investigation may give insights. Marc Van Gilst and Giana Angelo at the Fred Hutchinson Cancer Research Center in Seattle have demonstrated that during starvation, grown-up nematode worms can require propagation to be postponed pulverizing any current sex cells and recovering another yield of sound eggs from a couple of residual foundational microorganisms once conditions improve. Worms that experience this procedure additionally appear to stretch out their life expectancy up to triple. Van Gilst suspects that a flagging protein called NHR-49, definitely known to be associated with the metabolic reaction to fasting, is included: "In worms that contained an idle NHR-49 quality, regenerative recuperation and ripeness after starvation were seriously weakened," says Van Gilst.

From worm to human

He figures a comparable procedure that may exist in people. This is yet to be tried, in any case, and the trigger expected to actuate such a flagging pathway has not been distinguished. It may have advanced to enable our progenitors to save richness during times of starvation. One protein that may carry out the responsibility in people is called PPAR gamma, which is undifferentiated from NHR-49 and seems to control the pace of ovulation. It is likewise indistinct how much caloric limitation would be expected to turn on such a framework in people accepting we have it by any means. In any case, if the basic flagging atoms could be distinguished, and ways found to control them, it could help treat an assortment of ripeness issues and even broaden female regenerative life expectancy. On a very basic level, on the off chance that you can see how eggs start into the developing populace and you can back it off, at that point you would expand female ripeness.

Meal plans of intermittent fasting

IF, as we know is a style of eating where you abandon nourishment for a specific measure of time every day. To assist you with exploring your day, here is a manual on how to plan your dinners while fasting. Also, simply recall that this eating plan is organized around when you eat, what you eat too is as well significant. During the timeframes when you're eating, you'll need to concentrate on solid fats, clean protein, and starches from entire nourishment sources.

Step by step instructions to plan suppers when you doing IF.

While fasting can be overpowering, particularly on the off chance that you haven't done it previously, intermittent fasting can really be much simpler than numerous different sorts of eating plans.

When you start your intermittent fasting journey, you'll undoubtedly find that you feel more full and can keep the dinners you do eat basic. There are a couple of various ways you can quick, so I separated every one of the various plans beneath into basic, middle, medium and the advanced level. A common feast plan for your every day.

The mix of supplements will give you the vitality you have to improve the advantages of your fasting venture. Simply try to consider any individual nourishment bigotries, and utilize this as a guide for your specific wellbeing case, and change from that point. Keep in mind, that IF, doesn't really mean calorie-controlled, so be sure of what to eat as indicated by your own caloric needs.

1. The essential discontinuous fasting supper plan for learners.

On the off chance that you are an amateur, start by just eating between the long periods of 8 a.m. what's more, 6 p.m. is an extraordinary method to plunge your toes into the fasting waters. This arrangement permits you to eat each dinner in addition to certain tidbits yet get in 14 hours of fasting inside a 24-hour time frame.

Breakfast: Green Smoothie at 8 a.m.

In the wake of fasting, I like to slide into my day of eating with a smoothie since it is somewhat simpler for my gut to process. You'll need to go for a green smoothie instead of a high-sugar natural product smoothie to abstain from beginning your day on a glucose crazy ride. Include loads of solid fats to prop you up until lunch!

Fixings:

1 avocado

1 cup coconut milk

1 little bunch blueberries

1 cup spinach, kale, or chard

1 tablespoon chia seeds

Technique:

Include all fixings into blender, mix, and appreciate!

Lunch: Grass-Fed Burgers at 12 p.m.

Grass-took care of liver burgers are one of my preferred decisions for lunch during the week, and they are incredibly simple to prepare to have all through the whole week. You can eat this on a bed of dull verdant greens with a simple homemade dressing for a feast stuffed with B nutrients for solid methylation and detox pathways.

Fixings:

½ pound ground grass-took care of meat liver

½ pound ground grass-took care of meat

½ teaspoon garlic powder

½ teaspoon cumin powder

Ocean salt and pepper to taste

Wanted cooking oil

Strategy:

Combine all fixings together in a bowl and structure together wanted size patties.

Warmth cooking oil over skillet on medium-high warmth.

Cook burgers in skillet until wanted doneness.

Store in a compartment in the ice chest and use inside 4 days.

Bite: Cinnamon Roll Fat Bombs at 2:30 p.m.

Fat bombs will control your sweet tooth and give you enough sound fats to support you until supper, and these are particularly fulfilling in light of the fact that they suggest a flavor like cinnamon rolls.

Fixings:

½ cup coconut cream

1 teaspoon cinnamon

1 tablespoon coconut oil

2 tablespoons almond margarine

Technique:

Combine coconut cream and ½ teaspoon cinnamon.

Line a 8-by-8-inch square container with material paper and spread coconut cream and cinnamon blend at the base.

Combine ½ teaspoon of cinnamon with coconut oil and almond margarine. Spread over the main layer in the dish.

Freeze for 10 minutes and cut into wanted size squares or bars.

Supper: Salmon and Veggies at 5:30 p.m.

Salmon is a great wellspring of omega-3 sound fats, and dim green veggies like kale and broccoli are high in cell reinforcements. Salmon is one of my undisputed top choices for its taste and supplement thickness, however you can choose any wild-got fish based on your personal preference. Serve close by a portion of your preferred vegetables broiled in coconut oil, and you have a snappy and simple superfood feast.

Fixings:

1 pound salmon or other fish of decision

2 tablespoons new lemon juice

2 tablespoons ghee

4 cloves garlic, finely diced

Strategy:

Preheat stove to 400°F.

Combine lemon juice, ghee, and garlic.

Spot salmon in thwart and pour lemon and ghee blend over the top.

Wrap salmon with the foil and spot on a preparing sheet.

Prepare for 15 minutes or until salmon is cooked through.

In the event that your stove size permits, you can broil your vegetables close by salmon on a different heating sheet.

2. Middle of the road fasting supper plan

With this arrangement you will eat just between the long periods of 12 p.m. also, 6 p.m. for an entire 18 hours of fasting inside a 24-hour time frame.

I for one practice this arrangement during the week's worth of work. I'm not a morning meal individual, so I simply appreciate a couple of cups of natural tea to begin my day.

Despite the fact that you are skipping breakfast, it's as yet essential to remain hydrated. Make a point to in any case drink enough water. You can likewise have home grown tea, (Most specialists concur espresso and tea don't break your quick.) The catechins in tea have been appeared to improve the advantages of fasting by assisting with facilitating decline the yearning hormone ghrelin, so you can cause it until lunch and not to feel denied.

Since you've expanded your fasting period an additional four hours, you have to ensure your first feast (around early afternoon) has enough sound fats. The burger in the 8-to-6-window plan will function admirably, and you can include more fats in with your dressing or top with an avocado!

Nuts and seeds make incredible bites that are high-fat and can be eaten around 2:30 p.m. Splashing these in advance can help kill normally happening compounds like phytates that can add to stomach related issues. Have supper around 5:30 p.m., and simply like in the 8-to-6-window plan, a supper with a wild-got fish or other clean protein source with vegetables is an extraordinary alternative.

First dinner, 12 p.m.: Grass-took care of burger with avocado

Bite, 2:30 p.m.: Nuts and seeds

Second supper, 5:30 p.m :

Salmon and veggies

3. Propelled: The changed 2-day dinner plan

For this arrangement, eat clean for five days of the week (you can pick whatever days you need). On the other two days, limit your calories to close to 700 every day. Calorie limitation unlocks many of the equivalent benefits as fasting for a whole day. On your non-fasting days, you'll have to ensure you're getting in sound fats, clean meats, vegetables, and a few natural products, and you can structure your dinners anyway best works for you. On confined days, you can have littler suppers or snacks for the duration of the day or have a moderate-size lunch and supper and quick in the first part of the day and after supper. Once more, center around sound fats, clean meats, and produce. Applications can assist you with logging your nourishment and monitor your calorie consumption so you don't go more than 700.

Talk to your Doctor about a weight loss plan

Your Doctor assumes a significant job in your weight reduction achievement. Why? Since every health specialist can give basic data that may assist you with getting more fit. So set aside the effort to set up a date to work with your Doctor for weight reduction and diet help.

The initial phase in your weight reduction procedure will be to make a meeting with your doctor. Tell the assistant that you may require some additional time. At that point show up at your arrangement on schedule and set up a fair discussion about your wellbeing.

You may feel marginally awkward conversing with any health personnel or preferentially your doctor about your weight, yet do whatever it takes not to stress. Recall that your doctor is there to support you. On the note, that your weight is influencing your physical wellbeing, it's an ideal opportunity to desert shame and talk sincerely with the person in question. Plan to completely address any ailments that impact your eating regimen and any issues that can restrain your capacity to work out. You may likewise need to talk about clinical variables that may have caused weight gain.

At that point, prepare your inquiries. You may wish to record inquiries before you go and carry a pen and scratch pad to accept notes as you talk.

- Inquiries to pose include:

- Do I have to get more fit?

- What should my weight objective be?

- Are any of my wellbeing conditions identified with my weight?

- Am I in danger of creating different conditions as a result of my weight?

- Do any of the solutions I as of now take add to weight gain?

- Is there a weight reduction prescription ideal for me?

Notwithstanding these inquiries, you ought to likewise bring the subtleties of any eating regimen or exercise program you intend to begin. Your primary care physician can survey the arrangement for security and adequacy.

Best exercises to lose weight after 60

Exercise is considerably progressively powerful when matched with a sound eating regimen. There are a few difficulties to getting your wellness groove on after the age of 60: Both men and women experience age-related loss of slender tissue at this age, bringing about a more slow digestion and expanded muscle to fat ratio. That is the reason your fundamental objective ought to be concentrated on doing whatever you can to keep up and assemble muscle. This won't just improve your digestion yet it will set your body in the mood for maturing as restoratively as could reasonably be expected. Here, the four classes of activity you have to remain sound and fit at any age, in addition to how frequently you ought to do each kind of exercise.

Strolling

In addition to the fact that walking is an advantageous method to get in shape since you don't have to have a place with a rec center or put resources into unique hardware, it's likewise a perfect exercise for more established grown-ups since it's delicate on your joints and will help keep your heart and bones solid. A 155-pound individual consumes 149 calories when strolling at a moderate pace (3.5 mph) for 30 minutes, as indicated by Harvard Health Publishing. Increment the pace to 4 mph, and a similar individual consumes 167 calories. Obviously, running consumes more calories in a similar measure of time, yet strolling is a congenial, low-sway exercise that works for the vast majority. For steady weight reduction, youll need to time in at any rate 20 minutes of lively strolling most days of the week.

Lifting Weights

Lifting loads causes you to consume more fat, yet it likewise amps up your capacity to perform such day by day assignments as conveying staple goods, climbing stairs and doing other family unit tasks. Lifting loads is basic since we may all lose one to two percent of our muscle quality every year. Obstruction preparing with free loads is basic to shedding pounds, plus, solid leg and hip muscles lessen your danger of falling, a reason for significant inability among more seasoned grown-ups.

For lifting novices, we propose adequate and quality preparation at least two times each week, with exercises being part between chest area practices one day and lower body the other.

Tip: Skip the opposition machines and continue expanding the weight you're lifting when it turns out to be simple.

Yoga

In addition to the fact that yoga strengthens your muscles it builds your adaptability. Another advantage: Stretching and breathing profoundly during yoga assists with diminishing pressure hormones that add to midsection fat, a typical issue for anybody more than 60. Furthermore, since yoga lessens feelings of anxiety, it additionally can possibly improve your general dietary patterns (less pressure eating!), empowering weight reduction.

Interim Training

In case you're available, high-force interim preparing (HIIT), which is any exercise where you shift back and forth between extreme movement and less-exceptional action will assist you with consuming more calories. It's likewise one of the best approaches to get in shape, if you have your PCP's authorization for strenuous exercise. The best HIIT exercises for more established individuals simply beginning incorporate swimming and cycling. By doing to some degree hard interims followed by simple interims, you'll see huge enhancements in your high-impact wellness, quality and circulatory strain readings.

Looking younger without Botox, Laser and Surgery

We all wish to look way younger than our age, however, it we also don't want to go through botox, laser and surgery. There are numerous reasons why, including danger of inconveniences, dread of sedation, scars, and, potentially generally noticeable of all, cost. Truly, everybody can look ten years more youthful without having Botoxt, laser and medical procedure. You needn't bother with a facelift, eyelid lifts, or fat infusions to take look youthful. The following are basic strides to kick you off:

1. Lessening your sugar consumption - Multiple investigations have uncovered that sugar is the most horrible nourishment to eat for your skin. It ages the skin by making aggravation and through the procedure of glycation. So as to look more youthful and slow your skin's maturing, skirt sugary beverages and treats, and change from refined to entire grains.

2. Pick sound fats - Monounsaturated and polyunsaturated fats are known to alleviate the skin, decline irritation, and saturate the skin from the back to front. Wellsprings of these sound fats incorporate nuts, olive oil, avocados, and cold water fish (like salmon and fish). Attempt to stay away from nourishments high in soaked fats (like greasy cuts of hamburger, dull meat poultry, and particularly relieved meats like frankfurter and bologna) since these food sources can speed up your skin's maturing.

3. Eat brilliant products of the soil - Antioxidants are your body's best safeguard against free radicals. Free radicals are atoms that assault the solid cells of your body, including skin cells, making them be harmed and age all the more rapidly. Along these lines, eat nourishments wealthy in cell reinforcements, for example, vivid foods grown from the ground, to back off and even turn around the maturing procedure. This is an extraordinary motivation to visit your nearby ranchers' market!

4. Discard the cigarettes - Studies of indistinguishable twins have demonstrated that smoking cigarettes will make you age rashly. I see this in my office consistently. Smokers' skin is drier, not so much energetic, but rather more wrinkled than the skin of non-smokers. Despite the fact that stopping smoking won't turn around these progressions medium-term, it's the initial step that all smokers should take on the off chance that they would prefer not to age rashly.

5. Peel your skin 2-3 times each week - When we're youthful, our skin turns over each 6 two months. This procedure eases back as we age, making the upper layer of dead skin cells cluster superficially, making our skin look drier, show up progressively wrinkled, and feel more unpleasant in surface. Peeling the skin expels this upper layer of dead skin, uncovering the smoother, more beneficial skin beneath it. There are numerous approaches to peel, however the most effortless is to utilize a shedding clean that you can purchase at the medication store, or you can make one at home by joining heating pop, nectar, and milk.

A Typical schedule for the 16/8 method

IF is an eating plan on which you abandon nourishment for a specific measure of time. Furthermore, given the huge number of advantages (think weight reduction, glucose control, and even life span), it may not be an issue of whether you should attempt IF yet, rather which kind of irregular fasting to attempt. On the off chance that you are new to fasting, you likely need to begin with 16:8; because of its implicit adaptability and simplicity to follow.

How the 16:8 fasting plan functions.

The 16:8 fasting plan is an eating plan in which you embark on a fast for 16 hours every day and eat during an eight-hour window. This eating plan accompanies all the advantages of other fasting plans besides, late research finds that it might bring down circulatory strain. Maybe far better, you pick the eating window.

If you know you're not strong enough to do without breakfast, space your nourishment prior in the day (8 a.m. to 4 p.m.). On the off chance that you incline toward an early supper, eat in the day (11 a.m. to 6 p.m.). In case you're somebody who routinely goes out with companions for late suppers, plan your eating hours after the fact in the day (1 p.m. to 9 p.m.).

In spite of prominent attitude, there are no standards around what number of suppers you need to press in or whether you need to incorporate breakfast. Truth be told, no information really demonstrates the kind of breakfast that either makes you more beneficial or weighs less.

Instructions to begin with 16:8 fasting

When you settle on a general eating window and converse with an expert to ensure (IF) is directly for you, it's a great opportunity to bounce in however not really all in.

16:8 meal plan(sample)

Presently for the nourishment. Truly, 16:8 fasting gives you the opportunity to expend what you need during the eating window, however it is anything but a reason to go flapjack pizza-Pringles wild.

During your times of eating, you have to stay with a spotless, entire nourishments diet since a portion of the advantages of fasting incorporate decreased irritation, stacking up on shoddy nourishment during your eating window can sustain this aggravation. Also, with irritation being the basic contributing variable in practically all cutting edge medical issues, this is something you unquestionably need to monitor.

These implies yes to proteins, good fats, and sugars from entire nourishment sources. Skirt the ultra-processed nourishments and drive-through; simply don't avoid the attention on delectable. With less time spent on nourishment prep and arranging, it might even make you progressively inventive in the kitchen.

Here's a thought of what to eat (and when to eat it) on a 16:8 fasting diet, contingent upon which eating window you pick:

Early eating window meal plan

8 a.m: Egg and veggie scramble, side of entire grain toast

10 a.m: Yogurt and granola

12 p.m.: chicken and veggie pan sear

Night decaf tea

Late morning eating window dinner plan

Morning coffee or tea (zero sugar)

11 a.m.: Banana nutty spread smoothie

2 p.m.: avocado toast with pistachios

4 p.m.: Dull chocolate-shrouded almonds

6 p.m.: turkey meatballs and tomato sauce over entire wheat (or zucchini noodle) pasta

Late eating window supper plan

Morning dark espresso or tea (no cream or sugar)

1 p.m.: blackberry chia pudding

4 p.m.: dark bean quesadilla (cheddar of your decision, dark beans, ringer pepper, and taco flavoring)

6 p.m.: banana

9 p.m.: flame broiled salmon, vegetables, and quinoa

FAQ

Will eating my favorite meal break My Fast?

The absolute most posed inquiry! Fasting implies you are not eating. You can drink a few liquids however; these are the fluids to drink while fasting:

- Water
- Dark Coffee
- Green Tea, dark tea, other unsweetened tea

For whatever length of time that you're drinking one of these three things, you can drink as much as you need. Anything apart from this will trigger a type of insulin reaction.

Would i be able to drink Diet Soda while IF?

No you can't! Despite the fact that diet soft drink has zero calories, diet soft drink is more dangerous to your wellbeing than sugar-improved soft drinks. Don't put that bad, substance stuff into your body. An examination has indicated that diet soft drink may expand your insulin creation and may cause an expanded danger of unreasonable weight gain, type 2 diabetes and cardiovascular infection. We prefer you have a glass of water rather, if it's not too much.

Would i be able to drink Lemon Water on a Fast?

Sure! A tablespoon of lemon juice or Apple Cider Vinegar won't add enough calories to spike your insulin, so put it all on the line!

What are the Disadvantages of Intermittent Fasting?

Most impediments are quite minor and will leave following a little while. Here are two or three things individuals report when they attempt IF for the first time.

- Cerebral pains: Give it a little while, and these will typically leave.

- Numerous restroom trips: Only in light of the fact that you ought to drink a great deal of water during your fasting periods.

- You may feel cold, particularly your fingers: This is uplifting news on the grounds that your blood is heading out to your fat cells. The veins in your limits vasoconstrict to remunerate leaving you with cold fingers and toes.

Would i be able to Exercise during Intermittent Fasting?

Unquestionably! You can keep on practicing as you ordinarily do when fasting. In the event that you turn out hard while fasting you may see that your vitality levels are a piece lower, yet that is OK.

So, if you're a tip top competitor, converse with your mentor or nutritionist about your particular circumstance.

Will Intermittent Fasting Slow Down my Metabolism?

For quite a long time, we've been advised to eat at regular intervals. Three suppers and two or three snacks every day. In any case, by eating thusly, you never allow your body to consume something besides the nourishment you are eating. Intermittent fasting (IF) may, if not diminish your insulin levels so you begin loosing fat. Insulin advises your body to store fat and prevents your body from separating fat. So in the process of losing fat, you may end up diminishing your insulin levels. That is the reason this fasting is so viable.

Is Intermittent Fasting Safe for Women?

Women are quite complicated in their body system when it comes to Intermittent Fasting. No doubt animals and our science is the same. We bleed, ovulate, gestate, and lactate. We are an ensemble of hormones all doing various things at various phases of life. On the chance, that you are not worried about richness, IF is an extraordinary method to lose fat, get in shape and improve your wellbeing.

Would it be advisable for me to Cut Back on Calories for Extra Weight Loss?

Certainly not! Definitely slicing your everyday calories will hinder your digestion after some time. In the event that you keep on eating in a calorie shortage for an all-encompassing timeframe, your digestion will back off regardless of whether you are irregular fasting.

What advice would you give to anyone Intermittent Fasting?

- Drink water the entire day

- Remain occupied

- Try not to glut during your eating period

- Drink tea

- Never give-up: give (IF) at least a month.

- Eat well during your eating periods

- Attempt a low-carb diet to diminish appetite and make fasting simpler

Conclusion

There are many individuals getting incredible outcomes while following these techniques. Intermittent fasting (IF) isn't for everybody. It's not something that anybody needs to do. It's simply an instrument in the tool stash that can be valuable for certain individuals. Some additionally accept that it may not be as useful for women as men. It might likewise not be a prescribed decision for individuals who have or are inclined to dietary problems. Once you've made up your mind to attempt intermittent fasting, always bear in mind that you have to eat well too. It's unrealistic to gorge on lousy nourishments during the eating time frames and hope to get more fit and improve in wellbeing. There are lots of benefits accrued to Intermittent fasting if only done in the right way. With the information provided in this book, I know you are now ready to a step, achieving the very best for yourself.